# OXFORD MEDICAL PUBLICATIONS

WITHDRAWN

## THE FACTS

# ALSO PUBLISHED BY OXFORD UNIVERSITY PRESS

# Asthma

## THE FACTS
### Third Edition

· · · · · · · · · · · · · · · · · · · · · · · · · · · · · · · · · · · · · · · · · · · · · · · · · ·

BY

## DONALD J. LANE

*Consultant Physician, Osler Chest Unit*
*Churchill Hospital, Oxford*

Oxford   New York·  Tokyo
OXFORD UNIVERSITY PRESS
1996

Oxford University Press, Walton Street, Oxford OX2 6DP

Oxford   New York
Athens   Auckland   Bangkok   Bombay
Calcutta   Cape Town   Dar es Salaam   Delhi
Florence   Hong Kong   Istanbul   Karachi
Kuala Lumpur   Madras   Madrid   Melbourne
Mexico City   Nairobi   Paris   Singapore
Taipei   Tokyo   Toronto
and associated companies in
Berlin   Ibadan

Oxford is a trade mark of Oxford University Press

Published in the United States
by Oxford University Press Inc., New York

First edition 1979
Second edition 1987

A catalogue record for this book is available from the British Library

Library of Congress Cataloging in Publication Data

Lane, Donald J. (Donald John)
Asthma / Donald J. Lane. – 3rd ed.
Includes index.
1. Asthma–Popular works. I. Title II. Series. Facts (Oxford, England)
RC591.L34      1996      616.2 ' 38–dc20      95–52298
ISBN 0 19 262151 3

Typeset by Palimpsest Book Production Limited,
Polmont, Stirlingshire
Printed in Great Britain on acid-free paper by
Biddles Ltd, Guildford and King's Lynn

# Preface

It has become necessary to write a third edition of *Asthma: the facts*, not simply because the second edition had sold out, but because new knowledge has accumulated which needs to be more widely appreciated. Readers familiar with earlier editions will find some of the chapters reassuringly similar, but there are changes virtually throughout the book. We take a fresh look at the environment and highlight the problem of the rising prevalence of asthma. Important changes of emphasis in the treatment of asthma are covered and there is more detail in the sections dealing with the practical skills necessary to manage your own asthma.

Dr Storr's introduction on his experience as an asthmatic has been left intact. His asthma has become more stable. With the help of present day treatment, he has been able to lead an active life in retirement, much to the delight of those of us who enjoy the insights he brings to our understanding of human nature in his many books.

My life as a doctor has been immeasurably enriched by listening to asthmatics talk to me about their condition. Many of their experiences are reflected in the pages of this book. I have absorbed much too from the insights and discoveries of my colleagues working in basic science, clinical medicine, and nursing. To them we all owe a debt for their skills and devotion. My secretary, June Elsey, has faithfully transcribed my scribblings into a printable format and the staff at Oxford University Press have steered this third edition to the bookshelves. I thank them all.

I hope that those who enjoyed previous editions will pick up what is new in this rewriting, and that new readers will find much to interest them in the ever evolving story of asthma.

*Oxford*                                                                    D.J.L.
January 1996

# Contents

# Introduction

## Asthma as a personal experience

I first developed asthma in early childhood, though I cannot remember exactly what age I was when I had my first attack. Neither of my parents was asthmatic; but of their four children three suffered from asthma and other allergic disorders. My elder brother developed asthma in adult life when practising as a doctor in Devonshire; and the elder of my two sisters had to be removed from school on account of it. Only the younger of my sisters escaped. My elder sister also had infantile eczema and an allergy to fish. Two of my three daughters have shown allergies of different kinds; one to plants, the other to horses; the former has hayfever, the latter has had an attack of asthma. The asthmatic tendency has been passed on to my sister's grandchildren. This is a rather characteristic family history, except that it is surprising that neither of my parents showed any allergic tendency. However, they were first cousins; so it seems likely that they were carrying recessive genes predisposing to the disease which were made manifest in their children.

During my childhood, asthma was not nearly so serious a problem as it has become much later in my life. I suffered much more from hayfever, which made me dread the summer. Asthma used to accompany hayfever, and also occurred in association with colds. I was a sickly child who became accustomed to illness at an early age; and if I ever caught a cold or influenza, it would 'go to my chest'. Once I had bronchopneumonia but whether this made me more or less liable to asthma I cannot say. My earliest recollection of having asthma is of myself sitting up in bed leaning forward over a bed-table inhaling the smoke of 'Potter's Asthma Cure'. This was a powder containing stramonium (a drug which dilates the bronchi) which had to be ignited and which then emitted a smoke with a powerful and characteristic smell which comes back to me as I write. Potter's also made 'asthma cigarettes' containing the same powder. I have a vague recollection of smoking one of these and feeling very grown-up doing so; but I was not given them as often as the powder, which reminded me of one of those 'indoor' fireworks which one used to get out of Christmas crackers: a rather similar powder which also had to be ignited and which produced a long, snake-like shape when one set fire to it.

It is also characteristic of the allergic 'diathesis', that I should have had at least one attack of giant urticaria, which is popularly known as 'nettle-rash' and that I should have reacted excessively to insect-bites. When I was a child it was possible to write on my skin with a fingernail as red weals could be produced very easily. I am allergic to a number of different grass pollens, and still produce skin reactions to these when tested. I am also allergic to penicillin. Within minutes my skin became distended with fluid, and my face swelled to such an extent that I could pick up sections of it as if it was made of india-rubber. Fortunately this was in a hospital, and I was given an injection of adrenaline within a few minutes and quickly recovered. When I was thirteen I cut my head and developed a severe infection of the wound which rapidly led to infection of the bones of the skull and to a general septicaemia; that is, an infection severe enough for the bacteria causing it to be multiplying within the bloodstream. Today, this infection would have been cured within a few days by the administration of a suitable antibiotic; but, in 1933, even the sulphonamide group of drugs was not available, and I had to be given large doses of antistreptococcal serum to which, not unexpectedly, I had an allergic skin reaction.

My hayfever was treated by a long course of injections of 'Pollacine' which was developed in the laboratories of St Mary's Hospital as a way of desensitizing hayfever sufferers by giving them small but increasing doses of the pollens to which they were sensitive. I learned to give myself injections of this at the appropriate time of year, and persisted with them for several years. By the time I was about eighteen my hayfever was much less troublesome. I attributed this to the injections; but it is equally likely that the decline in severity was due to my having reached an age at which both hayfever and asthma often diminish or disappear, though why this happens is not known. Whatever the reason, I certainly lost both hayfever and asthma around that time, although I still became 'wheezy' if I caught a cold, and still developed irritation of the eyes during the summer even though I ceased to sneeze.

I cannot say that my childhood experience of asthma itself left any particular mark, for I did not have it nearly as severely as do many child asthmatics. On the other hand, it undoubtedly contributed to the picture which my parents and others had of me as 'delicate'. I was so often ill as a child that my parents decided that 'country air' would benefit me; and for this reason I was sent out of London to boarding school when I was eight years old. Like many other boys of my generation, I detested boarding school, and I am sure that the unhappiness I experienced there outweighed any possible benefit to my physical health. The effect of having asthma and other illnesses was to impair my physical confidence and to make me think of my body as a liability; a part of myself which I could not do without, but which was liable to let me down, and which was somehow inferior to those of other people. Freud rightly says that the ego is originally rooted in our physical being. I cannot remember a time when I liked my body or identified myself with it; it always seemed inefficient, or clumsy, or ailing. Physical confidence and confidence in other spheres go hand-in-hand; and my lack of physical confidence spread to include my abilities in general. Although I was for a time generally near the top of the class, by the time I was thirteen my performance deteriorated, and I did much less well throughout my school career than I should have. My impression is that many children who suffer a good deal of illness have the same experience. In my psychiatric work, I have generally managed to remember to enquire rather closely into my patient's history of physical illness in childhood, since I find that others have suffered in the same way as myself. Our adult psychological characteristics have roots in our childhood experience, and those who have a great deal of illness start with a disadvantage. However, a number of people react to this disadvantage as did Demosthenes to his stammer, or Franklin Roosevelt to his disablement by poliomyelitis. That is, they are driven to prove their worth by striving particularly hard to achieve something outstanding. Alfred Adler, who was originally an associate of Freud, but who parted from him to found his own school of 'Individual Psychology' laid emphasis upon how a particular physical weakness or 'organ inferiority', as he named it, could spur a person on to compensate or overcompensate, and thus achieve more than average in spite of a disability.

By the time I went to Cambridge – in 1939 – my health had improved, although I still became wheezy if I caught a cold. During my time at Westminster Hospital as a medical student I had an operation on my nose to remove a deflected nasal septum, the barrier down the middle of one's nose which separates the nostrils, and which is sometimes bent to one side or the other. I suspect that the fact that my nose so often became blocked was more due to allergic swelling of the mucous membrane than to the effects of a deflected septum; but the operation did something to relieve what had been a chronic problem. From 1939–69, however, I was almost free of asthma, although I continued to become wheezy to a very slight degree if I caught a cold, and always had a supply of ephedrine on hand to combat this. In 1969 asthma returned. Two factors may have contributed to this. First, I had another operation on my nose. By the end of 1968 I had lost my sense of smell altogether. Although this can in some circumstances be an advantage, the disadvantages outweigh the gains. One's sense of taste depends much more upon one's sense of smell than most people realize – one's actual taste buds only distinguish sweet, sour, salt, and bitter – and I could no longer enjoy food or drink in the way that I had done previously. The operation, known as an ethmoidectomy, cleared my nose of polyps, that is allergic swellings of the mucous lining of the nose, and my sense of smell was restored, at any rate partially. I later discovered that some authorities advise asthmatics against having nasal surgery unless it is absolutely essential on the grounds that it may make their asthma worse. However, there were no immediate effects from the operation, which was performed in the spring of 1969, and I cannot prove, though I strongly suspect, that it contributed to the return of asthma later that year.

The other factor which may have played its part was a period of stress which occurred in July and August of the same year. In 1968 a book of mine called *Human aggression* was published and achieved a modest success. On the strength of this I was invited to Harvard to give a course of lectures and seminars in their summer school. I had never taught undergraduates before, though of course I had taught doctors, nurses, social workers, and others in the course of my various appointments as a psychiatrist. Nor had I ever been to America. I remember arriving in Boston in intense heat – the temperature was in the nineties – which was accompanied by equally intense humidity. I took a taxi to the apartment I was renting from an art historian which was close to Harvard Yard. The apartment had been shut up for the past three weeks, with all the curtains drawn, and the temperature inside must have been about 103° Fahrenheit. I remember thinking that if this was what America was like I would have to go home. However, I succeeded in settling in and giving my two courses. One, which I much enjoyed, was to a small class of about twelve highly intelligent graduates on 'Creativity'. The other, which I dreaded, was to a class of about eighty undergraduates, on 'Aggression'. The lectures cannot have been a disaster, since I have been asked back to Harvard; but I cannot flatter myself that they were very good and I certainly felt tense and anxious during a good deal of the time I was in Harvard, although I also enjoyed a great deal of my stay, and made many new friends.

On my return, I went for a brief holiday to the Lake District. A third factor which may have contributed to the return of the asthma was that this particular house was ill-cared for and extremely dusty. However that may be, I developed a cough and wheeziness, and, to my horror, found that I could no longer walk as far as I had been accustomed to. Although never particularly robust, I had at least been able to walk; and, on my holiday in the previous year, had been able to walk twenty miles or more in a day in the mountains of Czechoslovakia.

At first, I did not believe that I had asthma, thinking that my cough and wheeziness was the result of bronchitis. But it soon became obvious that infection was not the prime cause, and I had to learn to accept the fact that, after thirty years of almost complete freedom from the disease, I was once again 'an asthmatic'.

As is common enough, my symptoms fluctuated in severity during that autumn. Then, in December 1969, I had a really bad attack. It so happened that, through no fault of his, my general practitioner could not be reached for a considerable time. I was in bed, panting away, wholly absorbed in the question of how I could get enough air into my lungs, although by this time my breathing was out of voluntary control and had become purely automatic. I began to realize that this attack was not only the worst attack of asthma which I had ever had myself, it was the worst attack that I had ever seen in anybody. Although I had been practising psychiatry for many years, I had, of course, treated asthmatics when I was a medical student and a house physician, and was familiar with attacks severe enough to warrant the patient's admission to hospital. As time went on, and the attack showed no signs of subsiding, I suddenly realized that I was in danger. I remember thinking to myself, 'If this goes on much longer, I might die'. At this point, I had a curious experience which has been reported before in those who have been close to death but lived to recount their story. I had what has been called an 'out-of-body experience'. That is, I became, as it were, detached from my own body, and almost seemed to be looking down on my heaving, panting frame from some point above it. At the same time, my anxiety and fear of dying was replaced by a sense of calm. I remember thinking,

'It might go either way. I wonder which way it will go. Perhaps this is the end of my life'. I did not find myself reviewing the events of my life, although I did think with regret that those dependent on me might find it more difficult to manage without me.

When my doctor finally arrived, he was clearly more anxious than I was myself. Fortunately, he carried oxygen in his car, and I was soon finding some partial relief by breathing it. He also gave me an injection of cortisone, and telephoned to the chest specialist whom I had consulted to enquire whether there was anything else he could do. Since he was an extremely experienced and conscientious doctor, there was, of course nothing else that the chest physician could suggest. I owe my friend Dr John Horder my life, and take this opportunity of thanking him, not only for saving me on this occasion, but for innumerable instances of devoted care over many years.

My 'out-of-body' experience is what psychiatrists call a 'schizoid' phenomenon. That is, it is an instance of a wider variety of phenomena which have in common the fact that, for the time, the person concerned is detached from the emotion which he would normally be expected to be feeling concurrently. If we are faced with something which is deeply painful or frightening, a protective mechanism comes into operation which prevents us being overwhelmed by grief or fear. Thus, a person who has been bereaved may, for a week or two, say that he feels numb or apathetic, and be unable to weep or show other signs of grief. A similar numbness often affects those who have been exposed to disasters like earthquakes. Sometimes those who have been through very disturbing experiences suffer from various symptoms like depression, anxiety, insomnia, and irritability which persist until they have been able to 'relive' the experience, and express the emotion connected with it which they were unable to express at the time; a phenomenon to which psychiatrists who treated battle casualties during the last war became accustomed. More often, the sufferer gradually works through his disturbing experience by repeatedly telling his friends about it until it seems to lose its emotional charge.

Although, like many asthmatics, I have from time to time had dreams of being drowned or stifled, I was not left with any severe after-effects from my experience of nearly dying, though it did leave me with a vivid realization that severe asthma is something to be taken seriously. It still seems to be a popular belief that people never die of asthma. In fact, some 2000 people in Great Britain die of it every year.

I have subsequently had a number of attacks of asthma, but only one has been as bad, or nearly as bad as this first really severe attack. This occurred while I was on holiday in Wales. My wife and I owned a cottage in a rather remote part of Wales on the borders of Snowdonia. We were there together when I developed severe asthma one evening which did not respond to treatment. My wife tried to summon help, but the telephone was out of order. By the time this was discovered, I was so bad that she did not like to leave me, nor did I wish for her to do so. We decided together that for her to fetch a doctor from the village was out of the question; and it also became obvious that I could not be driven to hospital as I was too ill to walk to the car, and she obviously could not carry me unaided. We therefore decided to stay together. Fortunately, when I felt that any breath might be my last, the spasm suddenly eased, and I started to recover. Experiences like this have taught me that it is wise to take precautions in advance, such as making sure that the telephone is working, and making contact with local medical facilities.

Since my asthma returned in 1969 I have been what is known as a severe chronic asthmatic. Although miracles sometimes happen, in this disease more than in others, I have no sustained hope of getting rid of it before my death. However, with the help of my doctors, Godfrey Fowler and Donald Lane, I have sufficiently mastered the disease for it to have become not entirely unreasonable to think that I might live long enough to die of something else. I now have much less time off work than I did when I first began to get bad attacks; although I may have to be away for a day or two when a bad attack first starts. I was admitted to hospital twice in the early part of 1976; but since then I have not been in hospital, which I attribute to my having learned something more about how to prevent attacks becoming out of hand. I therefore turn from a consideration of my own history to the problem of how to deal with asthma as a patient, in the hope that my experience may be of some use to others.

It has taken me a long time to learn how to cope with asthma at all effectively in spite of my medical training. One of the curious features of the disease, which others have noticed and commented upon, is a kind of false optimism between attacks. When asthma returns, it is natural enough to be somewhat depressed. Indeed, some observers believe that attacks of asthma are usually anticipated or accompanied by quite marked depression. I have not been sure that depression precedes an attack in my case, but I am sure that, once an attack is past, I am unrealistically euphoric and disposed to think that I may never have another. This extends to believing that, when asthma does start, it will not be very bad 'this time', and that I need not, therefore, take all the rather distasteful steps which are necessary to control it. This has meant that, in the past, I was reluctant to summon medical help even when the attack was obviously severe. I used to boast that I never allowed anyone to call the doctor until I was so breathless that I could no longer speak, but had to communicate in writing. I do not leave things so long today. A recent investigation in the Cardiff region showed that fatal attacks were typically short, lasting less than 30 minutes in 23 per cent and less than two hours in 25 per cent. It was also demonstrated that both patient and doctor were prone to underestimate the severity of the attack. I do not want to alarm my fellow sufferers, many of whom, although asthmatic, may never have had in the past or have in the future an attack with threatens life: but I do want to attack the conspiracy, to which asthma sufferers themselves contribute, which alleges that 'no one ever dies of asthma', and which contributes to unnecessary deaths by not taking severe attacks seriously. In Edinburgh, asthmatics who have previously been in hospital with severe asthma are encouraged to admit themselves to hospital without the need of medical referral. This probably saves a number of lives as, although there is no evidence from the Cardiff figures that there was any undue delay in the general practitioners getting to their asthmatic patients, it clearly saves time if the patient himself can initiate admission to hospital when necessary.

This brings me to another, most important aspect of coping with severe asthma. One is naturally reluctant to summon medical help unnecessarily, or to enter hospital unless it is absolutely essential, so that one is predisposed to treat severe attacks of asthma less seriously than is warranted. An interesting book on psychological factors in asthma by Aaron Lask, *Asthma: Attitude and milieu* (Tavistock, 1966), one of the many general practitioners trained in psychotherapy by the psychoanalyst Michael Balint, finds that the most severe asthmatics share an attitude of independence and reluctance to seek help. When Dr Lask and a group of his fellow practitioners started to investigate their population of asthmatics, they expected to find that a great many of them were demanding, using their illness as an excuse for getting attention and summoning the doctor when it was not necessary. In fact, though such patients existed, they formed only 15 per cent of the adult asthmatics in the practices investigated. Dr Lask found that most adult asthmatics managed their illness alone, and were reluctant to confide or to ask for help. I share this attitude. Moreover, however experienced one may be, it is extremely difficult to predict how severe any given attack is going to become. Sometimes, one may be severely breathless and noisily wheezy, and the attack will subside without progressing to anything alarming. At other times, an apparently less threatening attack will rapidly become severe. What is needed is an objective way of assessing the probable severity of an attack.

I have found that the use of a peak flow meter goes a long way to meeting this need. This is a device for measuring the rate at which one can force air out of one's lungs when one takes as deep a breath as one can, and then blows it out as fast as possible. If one blows into a peak flow meter, the needle records one's performance in litres per minute. As every asthmatic knows, breathing out is more difficult than breathing in; and the more the bronchi are obstructed by spasm and swelling, the more difficult it is to force air out of the lungs. Therefore, peak flow is a fairly objective measure of the degree of obstruction of the bronchi, and thus is a reliable indicator of the severity of the asthma. Since readings may vary slightly, it is advisable to take the best of three readings on any one occasion.

I have found that a great reduction in my peak flow often occurs *before* my asthmatic symptoms have become severe. In fact, I often refer to my peak flow meter as my early warning system. I have been in the habit of recording peak flow at the same time each morning and evening for a number of years, with the result that, by using appropriate drugs, I have been able to catch attacks at an early stage and prevent them from becoming too severe.

It is interesting to speculate as to why peak flow should be a better indicator of bronchial obstruction than one's own awareness of breathlessness. I think the answer is that, unless one has to climb stairs or run, one can suffer quite a large diminution in one's respiratory efficiency without being fully aware of how great that reduction is. If one is in good health, one does not realize what an enormous difference there is in one's requirements of oxygen when walking on the flat as compared with walking up stairs or running. Asthmatics soon become particularly aware of this discrepancy but, even so, can be deceived. When lying in bed or sitting still little oxygen is needed, and it is easy to be misled as to how difficult it may be to get more oxygen when that is required. I am sure I am not alone amongst asthmatics in having often woken in the morning with a conviction that an attack of asthma has almost subsided only to find that, when I get out of bed to empty my bladder, I am far more breathless than I had supposed. A peak flow meter will reveal the true state of affairs.

In my own case, a sudden drop in peak flow is a valuable warning sign, in exactly the same way as a drop in barometric pressure is a warning sign of rain to come.

The marked difference between readings in the early morning and readings in the early evening is not fully understood. If one is taking drugs for asthma, and takes the morning reading before having any medicines, as I do, the swing may be partly accounted for by the fact that the overnight gap between doses of medicine is the longest in the twenty-four hour period. Whatever the reason, my own peak flow, in between attacks of asthma, varies between 200 litres per minute in the morning and 300 litres per minute (or more if I am in particularly good form) in the evening. If the reading drops below about 140 litres I know I am in for trouble, and I am inclined to summon, or at least alert, my doctor. If it drops further, to about 120 or less, I am virtually immobilized; completely so if the reading is only 100. These figures are not to be taken as applying to anyone else; though we do have a clear idea of what is 'normal' in the average adult. It is simply to demonstrate that one's own, extremely shaky, unreliable subjective judgement can be reinforced by something much more objective which can provide a useful indication of what steps ought to be taken to both oneself and one's doctor.

I am quite sure that peak flow meters ought to be issued to all severe asthmatics. They are simple to use: and most patients can easily be taught to record morning and evening readings as I do.

From my own experience, and from what others tell me, I am certain that prevention in asthma is all-important. There is some curious mechanism, which we do not fully understand, which causes asthma to grow by what it feeds on. Although attacks cannot wholly be prevented, they can, to some extent, be anticipated; and the sooner remedial measures are begun, the less likely is the attack to become a bad one. Because asthmatics, as I have already mentioned, tend to be unrealistically optimistic, they often postpone taking steps to prevent an attack becoming severe, since they continue to hope that it will not become so. Asthmatics must learn to become self-medicators; to agree with their doctors what drugs are suitable in their particular circumstances, and to be familiar with the minimum and maximum effective doses of each. They will then be in a position to increase each drug to its permitted maximum whenever an attack threatens, reducing the dose if the attack passes off.

Severe attacks of asthma are alarming; and even if the thought of death itself is not necessarily threatening, inability to get enough air in and out of one's lungs is in itself a horrible, frightening experience, which provokes considerable anxiety. So much is this the case, that, in various parts of the world, mechanical interference with respiration is a well-known method of torture. In many prisons, those who are being interrogated have their heads plunged under water, which is often full of excreta, until they are nearly drowning. Another well-tried technique is to lie the victim down and pile slabs of stone on to his chest until it becomes more and more difficult for him to breathe at all. I can imagine exactly what such a prisoner feels. However, anxiety actually increases one's difficulty in breathing, and one can learn to control anxiety to some extent. Anxiety makes one breathe even more rapidly and shallowly than one needs; whereas exactly the opposite is required during a bad attack of asthma. Therefore, one must school oneself to breathe as deeply and slowly as is possible even while in the throes of an attack. One difficulty in doing this is that deeper breathing may make one cough; and coughing when the attack is at its height, makes one even more breathless. In a very severe attack, oxygen is often valuable. It is possible for doctors to prescribe oxygen under the NHS. I myself have a cylinder in my bedroom. Although I seldom need to use it, it is a comforting presence, and has in fact been invaluable on more than one occasion.

The anxiety which accompanies very great difficulty in breathing is also relieved to some extent by the presence of a loved one, and the touch of a loving hand. I feel no shame at all in recording that, when I have been desperately breathless, being able to grasp my wife's hand is enormously comforting.

When one is very breathless, to be able to sit up comfortably is very important. No asthmatic needs telling that his breathing is easier when he is sitting up than lying down; and most asthmatics will have their own arrangements of pillows which suit them. However, it is worth mentioning that it is easy to make a special bed-rest modelled on those huge cushions filled with plastic particles which were fashionable as substitutes for chairs some years ago. A smaller version of these has the advantage that, while it gives good support, it is also softer and more malleable than the ordinary bed-rest. However, bed itself is not a comfortable place for asthmatics, since it is easier still to breathe if one's legs are hanging down. So sitting in a suitable chair, provided one can be kept warm, is still more comfortable. The idea that one must be 'in bed' if very ill is difficult to dispel; but I think that it is easier to manage asthma oneself if one is sitting up in an armchair.

During a bad attack of asthma one's appetite usually disappears entirely. Moreover, eating generally makes one's breathlessness worse. However, one has to try and eat something, at least when the attack is beginning to subside, and my own experience has led me to believe that little and often is far better than having a large meal. It is extremely important, however bad one is, to drink large quantities of fluid; and it will be found that to do so does not increase, and may diminish, the severity of the symptoms. I find that lime juice or lemon barley water encourages me to drink more than I would if I confined myself to water which, in cities in Britain, is often so heavily chlorinated as to taste extremely unpleasant. The reason that one ought to drink as much fluid as possible during asthma is that one becomes dehydrated during a bad attack. There is some evidence that the extreme stickiness of the sputum, which constitutes one of the most tiresome features of asthma, is reduced if one imbibes enough fluid.

Sleep is always a problem during the course of a bad attack of asthma. It is always disturbed, and one may only be able to doze intermittently throughout the night. It is important not to take any kind of sleeping pill, since nearly all such medicines tend to depress respiration still further. I have found, however, that a very small quantity of whisky enables me to get some sleep without having any adverse effect that I can detect.

If one has a sleeping partner, problems may arise. On the one hand, a bad attack of asthma may demand immediate help; unscrewing the nut on the oxygen cylinder, for instance; or telephoning the doctor if the attack gets worse. On the other, knowing that one is keeping one's partner awake increases one's own anxiety and distress. In the house I live in, we have solved the problem by my wife being able to sleep in a bedroom immediately opposite to the one we usually share. We both leave our doors slightly ajar; and I have a small handbell which I can ring if things get desperate. This works very well, as I prefer to be alone when having asthma in order to be free to cough, move in bed, put the light on and so on without disturbing anyone else.

It is also a great advantage if the room in which one sleeps is on the same level as a lavatory. I share the dislike of bedpans and bottles which most patients have; and if I can manage to totter to a lavatory during even a bad attack of asthma, I do so.

When a bad attack of asthma subsides, it is important to take things slowly and easily. Objective tests show that one's blood gases and metabolism take time to get back to normal; and a bad attack leaves one exhausted for a while.

The main problem of the aftermath, at any rate in my case, is to get rid of the accumulated sticky sputum which is such a feature of asthma, and which, in fatal cases, is the cause of death by plugging the smaller air passages. I think it is important to clear one's lungs of this as fast as possible: for my private, unsubstantiated belief is that the more mucus which remains in the bronchial tree, the more does it act as an irritant provoking both the production of still more mucus, and also bronchoconstriction. During a bad attack of asthma, coughing may have to be suppressed, since it sometimes increases breathlessness to an intolerable degree. When the attack is subsiding, I find that coughing is often far less helpful in getting rid of sputum than I would like it to be. I think this is because coughing tends to constrict the bronchi still further, which makes it impossible for the sputum to be expelled. I have found it useful to breathe out against slight resistance: that is, by pursing one's lips as if one was going to whistle and then breathing out in a slow and determined fashion. This technique helps to bring up sputum to the point at which it can gently be coughed up without difficulty. Another valuable way of hurrying mucus up the bronchial tree is to blow one's nose gently. It is important to avoid violent coughing as much as possible since this is not only exhausting, but also may damage one's lungs.

When physiotherapy is available, this is often helpful in speeding up the process of clearing one's chest of accumulated secretion. Physiotherapists often use a 'Bird' respirator which blows humidified oxygen into one's lungs. This can help one to clear out the loosened sputum by a combination of techniques of 'assisted respiration' and 'postural drainage'.

Although, as a medical student, I was taught that expectorant drugs were largely useless, research has shown that some drugs do accelerate the passage of mucus up the bronchial tree. I use a preparation containing guiaphenesin.

I am also a believer in the old-fashioned remedy of 'inhaling'. It probably does not matter whether one uses Friar's Balsam or one of the modern, proprietary capsules which have largely replaced it, since it is likely to be steam, rather than whatever is added to it which is helpful. However, I have found that sticking one's head over a jug of boiling water with some reasonably pleasant-smelling medicament in it does seem to loosen sputum and make it easier to expel. The smell of eucalyptus is difficult to get rid of; and so I use a special jug for inhaling. Plastic jugs which withstand boiling water are now available, and seem very suitable. So much for dealing with the attack.

In between attacks I try to be a 'good patient' and obey my doctors' instructions. That is, I take the drugs which they tell me to take, although it is a nuisance never to be able to travel anywhere without carrying two different aerosols and a variety of tablets. Although I am not taking oral steroids all the time, I do have to take large doses when an attack starts; and, by the time I have reduced the dose to nil, I generally have only a week or two before the next attack occurs. I dislike having to take steroids because, like many other people, I dislike being dependent on drugs which interfere with the roots of my emotional being and also alter my facial appearance. One's hormonal system, unlike one's stomach or kidneys, is intimately connected with one's self and one's emotional responsiveness. I haven't suffered severely from the emotional disturbances which are described in some patients who have to take steroids, apart from one short-lived attack of depression: but I confess to a feeling of unease that these powerful drugs may not only relieve asthma but alter my personality.

Although my capacity for physical exercise is now impaired, I do try to take some, and also try not to put on weight; a tendency which is enhanced by steroids. Large meals tend to make me wheezy, and so I usually avoid them. Some forms of alcohol seem to provoke asthma; but whisky seems the least provoking of alcoholic drinks, and I drink this in preference to other forms of alcohol.

As a psychiatrist, I shall be expected to say something about psychological factors in asthma, which is often labelled a 'psychosomatic' disease. When I was a medical student, it was fashionable to suppose that asthma, duodenal ulcer, ulcerative colitis, hypertension, and a few other diseases were primarily the result of emotional conflicts. In Chicago, the psychoanalysts Alexander and French thought that they had pin-pointed the psychological cause of asthma, amongst other diseases. They believe that asthma took origin from a particular conflict, starting in childhood, which consisted of a deep dependence upon the mother or mother-substitute combined with a fear of becoming estranged from her by somehow offending her. In *Psychoanalytic therapy* they quote a case of a young man whose asthma was relieved by psychotherapy when he came to realize that his dependence upon his stepmother was compli-cated by sexual desires toward her. In other cases, it was supposed that the child had aggressive feelings toward his mother which he dared not express for fear of losing her support. There are two difficulties about this kind of explanation. One is that the number of cases described is minute, so that there is really no evidence that the explanation invoked fits more than a tiny minority. The other is that, especially in the case of psychosomatic disorders, the psychopathology which is postulated is generally concerned with conflicts and impulses which are universal. What human being, in childhood, has not had conflicts between dependence and independence? Which of us have not felt aggressive towards those upon whom we are dependent? The hope that any given psychosomatic disorder has a specific emotional conflict at the root of it has not been fulfilled. Indeed, many of us have given up using the term 'psychosomatic' in the belief that it is a cloak for ignorance rather than a description of any value. This is not to say that stress is incapable of precipitating asthma, or of making it worse once it is established. In my career as a psychiatrist I remember one case of asthma, though only one, in which I felt certain that stress had played the major part in initiating the disease. This was the case of a lady who had her first attack of asthma in middle age, and who went on to become a severe asthmatic. Before the asthma started she had been subjected to considerable stress in that her husband had developed a premature form of senility due to brain disease (presenile dementia). Since he was incapable of earning, his wife had had to take on the responsibility of going out to work for the first time in her life in order to meet the rather heavy financial commitments which the family had shouldered. That her asthma was directly connected with her husband's collapse was demonstrated by her dream that she was tightly wrapped in a carpet whilst he sat on her chest, making it almost impossible for her to breathe. Such cases are, however, rare; and I do not think that stress of this kind is often a suf-ficient, although it may be a subsidiary, factor in provoking asthma.

Various investigations have been undertaken in the hope of discovering an asthmatic personality; but there is little evidence that such a thing exists. Some asthmatics are neurotic; others are not; and when asthmatics do show neurotic traits, it is hard to decide whether these traits are a cause or a result of the disorder. There is, however, some consensus of opinion that asthmatics are over-controlled and tend to bottle up their emotions. Dr Lask and his colleagues, whose work I referred to earlier, found that the majority of asthmatics were reluctant to ask for help, but that the minority who made many demands upon their doctors tended to have attacks of asthma which were less severe. This finding might be interpreted as evidence that asthmatics are essentially rather dependent people but are reluctant to admit or to give in to this aspect of their personalities. This interpretation is supported by one study which found that in Maryland, asthma was more commonly found in boys from middle-class families in which particular emphasis is laid upon achievement and independence. In dealing with my own asthma I have learned that to try to maintain too stiff an upper lip is a mistake, in that it is better to seek help early rather than later.

However, there is no doubt that emotional stress has an effect upon asthma once it is established, although it is difficult to predict whether emotional arousal will make asthma worse or better. The physician Sir Arthur Hurst once had an attack of asthma while driving. He fumbled a gear change and found himself speeding down a hill in neutral with the car out of control. By the time he had reached the bottom of the hill his asthma had disappeared. Hurst supposed that his anxiety had caused his adrenal glands to produce more adrenaline, which thus relieved his asthma; but anxiety does not invariably have this effect. I can recall two instances in my own case in which anxiety made asthma worse. One was when I thought that a hotel had overcharged me, and that I should have to dispute the bill, a thing which I very much dislike having to do. The other was when I was in charge of my two-year-old grandson when he slipped and cut his head. As soon as I had taken him in to his mother and made sure that he was not badly injured my wheeziness subsided. The fact that asthma can be made worse or relieved by emotional arousal does not imply that the cause of asthma is primarily emotional. It is hard to think of any physical condition which is not influenced by the patient's emotional state, from headache to rheumatoid arthritis. However, if stress does play a part in inducing asthma, I suggest that our failure to have discovered a more clearcut relationship between supposed cause and effect may be due to the fact that stress has effects which may not be manifested for years after the event. We know that people who have been in concentration camps suffer both in physical and mental health for years afterwards; probably for the rest of their lives. But we do not yet know in detail how the effects of stress are mediated. The endocrine system, particularly, is enormously complicated; and, although advances in understanding are made every year, we are still ignorant about many features of its functioning. I am quite prepared to believe that my personality and that of other asthmatics is related to peculiarities in the endocrine system and those physiological functions which are concerned with defence against disease. But I think that, in our present state of ignorance, it is premature to make any generalizations about personality characteristics or neurotic traits in any so-called psychosomatic disease, including asthma.

I will not pretend that asthma is anything but a liability which I would much rather be without. However, whenever I am inclined to be sorry for myself, I think of those who have to cope with chronic illnesses which are far, far worse, like multiple sclerosis. Thanks to a great deal of expert, devoted help from my colleagues, I have learned to cope and to live with asthma; and I look forward to the day when the underlying cause of this common disease will be better understood than it is today.

The following chapters depict the facts about asthma as they are known today. Greater understanding has, in my case, helped me to live with asthma and overcome many of the problems associated with it. I hope that others may be able to benefit as I have.

## Addendum

Since this book was first published in 1979, there have been some innovations in treatment which I have found helpful. The first is the 'Nebuhaler'. This is a plastic container (see p. 164) for use with aerosol sprays. It has been shown that delaying and spacing out the dose from a pressurized aerosol enables more of the dose to reach the lung. Aerosols often have such a powerful propellant that a good deal of the drug is lost by being deposited in the mouth and throat, since it is difficult to time one's intake of breath accurately to coincide with the operation of the aerosol spray. By giving a little more time, the use of 'Nebuhaler' ensures that the patient inhales a greater proportion of the dose delivered by the aerosol.

Another, very important innovation is a pressurized nebulizer. When a patient is severely asthmatic, the inflow and outflow of breath (tidal volume) may be so small that it is very difficult for him or her to inhale any medication at all, even from a pressurized aerosol. His bronchi are so blocked with mucus and by spasm that very little air or medicine can get in and out. A nebulizer, used with a special solution of one or other of the bronchodilating drugs like salbutamol, creates a fine mist in which the drug is suspended in very small particles. These particles are able to enter the bronchial tree much more effectively than those from a conventional aerosol.

I possess a type of nebulizer which will either plug into the ordinary electricity supply, or which will run off a car battery. It will also easily convert for use in countries which use a different voltage. If I am on my travels, I always take it with me, and it has been extremely valuable on several occasions. It is not for routine use, nor is it a replacement for other forms of treatment. No one who is on steroids, for instance, should think that, because he has a nebulizer, he need not bother to take steroids or increase the dose when necessary. But, in a severe attack of asthma, there is no doubt that the use of a nebulizer can be invaluable.

In conclusion, since this is a personal, rather than a medical chapter, I would like to inform my readers that, on the whole, I have continued to manage asthma with increasing skill, and have avoided any further hospital admissions for the disease. However, I have experienced one extremely alarming and sudden attack which came on quite unexpectedly. I was walking through the West End of London, so confident that I was free of asthma that I had no medicines with me, not even an aerosol spray. I rapidly became extremely disabled. Fortunately, I was able to get a taxi to take me to the garage where my car was parked, and in the car was my nebulizer and other drugs. I just managed to plug the nebulizer into the car battery, and soon began to recover. Looking back, I think I should have asked the taxi driver to take me to hospital. The moral of this story is that, however well an asthmatic seems to be, he or she should never, never venture anywhere without taking at least an aerosol spray in bag or pocket. Asthma can come on with unpredictable speed and intensity, and such attacks are dangerous.

I would like to thank all those readers who have written to me about this personal account, and to wish my fellow-asthmatics the best of both skill and luck in managing their disability.

# Defining asthma

# 1 What is asthma?

Asthma is a condition which is easy to recognize, yet difficult to define. There can be few who have not seen the attacks of wheezy laboured breathing that are the hallmark of asthma. It commonly afflicts the young, though they frequently grow out of it. When it starts or reappears later in life, it tends to persist into old age. Death from asthma is uncommon, but not so infrequent that either doctors or patients can be complacent.

Difficulties in defining asthma are twofold. First, the chief symptoms of asthma—wheezing, cough, and breathlessness—all occur, separately or together, in other chest conditions. And secondly, whilst it is a characteristic of asthma that these symptoms are variable rather than constantly present, getting agreement on the degree of variability that justifies the label 'asthma', has proved contentious. So it is not perhaps surprising that when a group of experts sat down to *define* asthma in 1972 they came to the conclusion that on the evidence currently available they could not do so. Yet each freely admitted to the others, that they could readily *recognize* asthma when they saw it.

## A brief history

These perplexities can perhaps be better understood by taking a historical perspective. The word asthma is Greek. It meant panting and was one of the words coined to describe shortness of breath. Laboured and difficult breathing was called dyspnoea, '*dys*' meaning difficult, and '*pnoea*' meaning breathing. Breathing difficulties when lying flat were orthopnoea; '*ortho*' meaning straight or flat. These two words are still in use and so, of course, is asthma. From the very beginning it signified a breathing difficulty that, although alarming when it happened, came only sporadically.

Some of the most eloquent descriptions of asthma come from Aretaeus the Cappadocian in the second century AD. 'The lungs suffer and the parts which assist respiration sympathize with them.' He wrote of the rapid noisy breathing of the asthmatic and of the anxiety and fear it induced. 'They eagerly go into the open air, since no house sufficeth for their respiration.'

The accurate observations of Aretaeus were lost for over a millenium while medicine lay under the influence of Galen. Born at Pergamon in Asia Minor in AD 131, Galen dominated medical thought for centuries. Sadly he completely misunderstood the function of the lungs and heart and had little of worth to offer on asthma. The Arabian physician Rhazes remarked, 'Galen said that many cure asthma with owl's blood given in wine. I say that owl's blood is not to be given, for I have seen it administered and it was useless'. Wisdom, too, can be found in the words of the great physician of Western Islam, Moses Maimonides. During the twelfth century, just as the sun was setting on Arabic influence in Europe, he taught that the patient must be treated as a whole and humbly recognized his therapeutic limitations. 'This disease has many aetiological aspects . . . it cannot be managed without a full knowledge of the patient's constitution as a whole . . . furthermore I have no magic cure to report.'

Often an illness is seen in a new light when the physician is himself the sufferer. Two English physicians in the second half of the seventeenth century wrote at length and sensibly about asthma. Thomas Willis and Sir John Floyer. Willis viewed asthma as alarming: 'There is scarce anything more sharp or terrible than the fits thereof.' Though his ideas on lung function were firmly Galenic, his observations have a curiously modern flavour. 'Whatsoever, therefore, makes the blood to boyl or raises it into an effervescence, as violent motion of the body or mind, excess of intern cold or heat, the drinking of wine, venery, yea sometimes mere heat of the bed, doth cause asthmatical assaults to such as are predisposed.'

Floyer suffered under the 'tyranny' of asthma for thirty years. 'The asthma is a laborious respiration with lifting up the shoulders and wheezing . . ., 'tis observed that the asthmatic cannot cough, sneeze nor speak easily, because a sufficient quantity of air cannot be drawn into the lungs to produce those actions.' The 'pipes of lungs' had been described by this time and there was an awareness that these air passages, the bronchi, were implicated in asthma. Floyer wrote: 'I have assigned the immediate cause of the Asthma to the straightness, compression or constriction of the Bronchi', and Willis wrote that asthma was due 'to cramps of the moving fibres of the bronchi.'

It is interesting to reflect that when John Floyer and Thomas Willis were writing about asthma, they had no idea of the true function of the

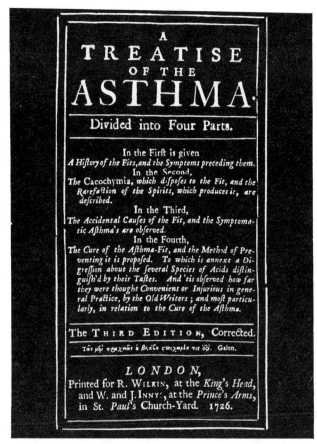

A

# TREATISE

### OF THE

# ASTHMA.

### Divided into Four Parts.

In the Firſt is given
*A Hiſtory of the Fits, and the Symptoms preceding them.*
In the Second,
*The Cacochymia, which diſpoſes to the Fit, and the
Rarefaction of the Spirits, which produces it, are
deſcribed.*
In the Third,
*The Accidental Cauſes of the Fit, and the Symptoma-
tic Aſthma's are obſerved.*
In the Fourth,
*The Cure of the Aſthma-Fit, and the Method of Pre-
venting it is propoſed. To which is annext a Di-
greſſion about the ſeveral Species of Acids diſtin-
guiſh'd by their Taſtes. And 'tis obſerved how far
they were thought Convenient or Injurious in general Practice, by the Old Writers; and moſt particularly, in relation to the Cure of the Aſthma.*

The **THIRD EDITION**, Corrected.

Τῶν μὲν πϱαχυὰτ ὁ βλάζα ϛυνχωϱία τις ὄϑι. Galen.

### *LONDON,*

Printed for R. WILKIN, at the *King*'s *Head,*
and W. and J. INNY:, at the *Prince*'s *Arms,*
in St. *Paul*'s Church-Yard. 1726.

The frontispiece to Floyer's book on asthma

lungs. They believed, like their predecessors, that air was drawn into the lungs to cool the blood. Not until the second half of the eighteenth century did Lavoisier conclusively demonstrate that a gas, named by him oxygen, was removed from the air by breathing and that this gas was essential to life.

## How the lungs work

We have the advantage over our eighteenth-century predecessors in possessing a very detailed knowledge of the structure and functioning of our bodies. It will be helpful at this stage to look a little more closely at the way in which the lungs are constructed and the way in which they work. One lung is situated on each side of the chest. Each has a sponge-like structure. The spaces in the sponge—there are about 300 million of these—connect to the outside through a series of branching pipes through which the air passes. Blood is supplied to the lungs from the right side of the heart and returned to the left side of the heart.

The lungs fill most of the space within the chest. A slight vacuum holds them out against the inner wall of the rib cage. Air is drawn into the lungs and expelled from them by the action of muscles in the chest wall. The muscles between the ribs widen the rib cage when breathing

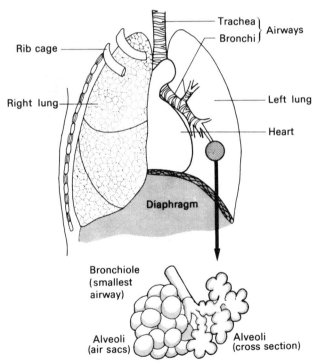

The lungs showing how they are situated inside the chest, with some details of the airways and air sacs.

in and narrow it during breathing out. Beneath the lungs lies the most important muscle for breathing, the diaphragm. When it contracts it pulls downwards, sucking air into the lungs. When it relaxes, the lungs recoil back to their resting position.

The muscles of breathing are unique amongst the body's musculature. They can be moved at command but also operate automatically. We can fill our lungs full of sea air. We can hold our breath to keep out smoke. We can shout or sing. The use of the muscles of breathing in these ways is akin to the use of arm or leg muscles for writing or walking. But whereas arm and leg muscles remain stationary unless we will them to move, the muscles of breathing do not. They have an automatic or involuntary rhythm of their own. Whether we are dozing in a chair or running for a bus, the muscles of breathing keep up their regular movement. In this respect they are behaving like the muscles of the heart. Heart muscle action is, however, almost wholly automatic and we have very little, if any, voluntary control over it. So the unique nature of the muscles of breathing lies in their dual control, for the most part automatic, but available for voluntary use.

The purpose of breathing is to move air in and out of the lungs. From the incoming air, oxygen is transferred to the blood to be pumped around the body by the heart. From the blood, carbon dioxide—the waste gas produced from the use of the oxygen—is transferred to the air in the lungs and so breathed out. By ingenious devices which detect the level of both the oxygen and carbon dioxide in the blood, the brain regulates the degree and rate of movement of the chest, so that just the right amount of oxygen is supplied for the moment-to-moment needs of the body. In sleep, breathing is slow and shallow because little oxygen is required. In exercise, large quantities of oxygen are needed: so breathing is rapid and deep.

Air enters the lungs through a single tube, the trachea or windpipe. The trachea is some 10–12 cm long and about 2 cm wide. It branches into two main air passages—the major bronchi—which supply the right and left lungs. Division then continues more or less regularly 10 to 25 times ending with thin flexible tubes of about half a millimetre bore. Off these, 300 million air sacs, or alveoli, bud, so that their external appearance is very much like bunches of grapes. The internal surface of these numerous air sacs is vast, sufficient if spread out to cover an area about the size of a tennis court.

The blood vessels supplying the lungs also divide up from a single supply vessel but in nothing like so regular a fashion. They branch into a myriad of tiny thin-walled capillaries coursing over the surfaces of the air sacs. Through the thin walls of the alveoli, the blood in the capillaries picks up oxygen and gives off carbon dioxide, and returns, replenished to the heart.

## The airways in asthma

It is with the airways, or bronchi, that the trouble lies in asthma. The air sacs are spared and if air gets to them they behave normally. *If* the air gets to them; for in asthma it may fail to do so. In asthma there is narrowing or even blockage of the bronchi. As a result great effort is required to draw air in and out of the lungs. When the air is forced through a narrow airway, it produces a whistling or wheezing sound rather like blowing a wind instrument.

Bronchial narrowing may be caused in several ways: by mucus poured into the bronchi, by swelling of the internal layers of the bronchi, or by contraction of muscle lying in the walls of the bronchi which leads to constriction of the air passages. These three mechanisms for narrowing the airways need to be looked at in greater detail.

Like most surfaces of the body, the bronchi have several layers. The lining layer, known as the bronchial mucosa, is very thin. Its surface cells point inwards. They are lined by extremely fine hairs. These hairs, or cilia, beat in rapid motion up towards the mouth carrying with them a thin layer of mucus. Particles of dust inhaled into the lungs are caught up in the mucus layer and so are carried by the wafting action of the cilia

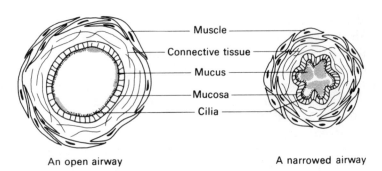

An open airway                              A narrowed airway

The detailed structure of the airways.

away from the deeper parts of the lung. The mucus itself is produced by other cells in the lining layer, some of which are collected together in clusters, the mucous glands. One of the ways in which narrowing of the airways occurs in asthma is by an excess of mucus produced in response to inflammation of the lining of the airway.

The lining cells sit on a layer of rather nondescript tissue which acts as a packaging material. It is a tissue that lies beneath many body surfaces and which allows a certain amount of movement. Pick up a piece of skin over the back of the hand, for example, and you will find you can move it backwards and forwards over the underlying muscles and bones. A similar flexibility exists beneath the surface layers of the bronchi. Because this is a loose layer of tissue, it can readily become swollen. Thinking again of the skin; after a bee sting, a swelling appears. This consists mostly of fluid derived from the blood. Swelling of the tissues beneath the lining layer of the bronchi occurs during asthma. It is another cause of narrowing of the airways. In the severest asthma attacks, this swelling can be so great that it pushes the surface lining off. This, in combination with thick sticky mucus, can produce a plug which actually blocks the airway, rather than just narrowing it.

Throughout most of the airways there is beneath these linings a muscle layer. The strands of muscle wind spirally around the airway so that when they contract they squeeze the airway and so narrow it.

Contraction of bronchial muscle occurs in asthma. It can be the sole factor causing airway narrowing. In this case, the change in calibre is usually short-lived, perhaps lasting only a minute or so. It more often occurs together with swelling and mucus production to cause a more persistent airways narrowing lasting several hours. Contraction is not quite the appropriate word for this prolonged shortening of muscle, and the term bronchospasm has been used. In the past too much emphasis has been laid on bronchospasm as a cause of bronchial narrowing leading to the neglect of other components such as swelling and mucus. Much is now known about the production of mucus and the cause of the swelling. As we shall see later, this has resulted in effective remedies designed to relax narrowed airways.

## So what is asthma?

We are now in a position to formulate an answer to the question posed at the heading of this chapter 'What is asthma?' Asthma is a condition in which there are episodes of breathing difficulty due to widespread narrowing of the airways of the lungs. This narrowing can be due to mucus in the airway, to swelling of the lining of the airway, or to spasm of the muscle in the walls of the airways, or to a combination of all three.

It may be questioned whether asthma should be regarded as a disease in its own right, or whether it is merely a symptom of one or several other disorders. This hinges very much on defining the word disease. Taken in a colloquial sense, it implies a state of disturbance: disturbance from what is generally regarded as normal; indeed disturbance in a disadvantageous direction. The description of a disease begins with symptoms, the reporting of what brings dis-ease. The physician, basing his observations on many patients, will try to work out what changes in the body are responsible for this state of disease. Finally, working with his scientific laboratory colleagues, the physician will, it is hoped, be able to identify a cause for the bodily disturbance.

This approach can be applied to any disease. A simple example is the complaint of a sore throat. On a symptomatic level the disease is simply that: a sore throat. In anatomical terms 'throat' would be translated into Greek to describe the part involved: the pharynx. To describe the functional abnormality, namely inflammation, the ending, 'itis' is added, so giving the combination: 'pharyngitis'. If laboratory tests demonstrate an infection in the throat, such as the bacterium Streptococcus, a full description can be packaged into the term 'Streptococcal pharyngitis'.

How far this analysis can be applied to asthma will become apparent throughout this book. The symptomatic description is satisfactory and can be condensed into 'episodic wheezy breathlessness'. The site of the disease is the lungs and the all important change is to do with narrowing of the air passages. The reasons why this narrowing occurs are various and it will emerge later that even in a given individual, it may not be possible to pin-point a single cause for asthma. Asthma in this sense can be looked upon as an abnormal pattern of behaviour of the airways, which has many causes or triggers. This will lead us to think in terms of some underlying disturbance in the airways which renders them liable to behave in this way.

The advantage of regarding asthma in this way is that it enables us to examine the same phenomenon—'episodic wheezing'—in large numbers of people and hopefully draw some conclusions as to why it occurs. The disadvantage is that it obscures what happens in individuals. We shall explore this in more detail later but briefly we shall find that the individual, who at one time has clearly defined episodic wheezing, may at other times have coughing only, may enjoy prolonged spells of months or years without symptoms, or may, unfortunately, become progressively and permanently short of breath. Describing such an individual's lifetime of symptoms as 'asthmatic' broadens the definition of the word to such an extent that it might be preferable to have a different label (or labels) to describe the whole pattern of disease in the individual. This has not yet been done in any consistent way and the word 'asthma' is still used quite loosely, both to describe the pattern of behaviour that is just episodic wheezing and also the lifetime of symptoms in given individuals who therefore have asthma as a disease.

## ... And what is not asthma?

It is worthwhile at this stage disposing of one or two other words which are either used in connection with asthma, or get confused with it. The word 'asthma' was till recently attached to the breathing difficulties experienced by some patients with heart diseases. 'Cardiac asthma' is a quite separate problem from 'true asthma' or 'bronchial asthma' so that most physicians have dropped the term. When used as a word on its own, asthma means bronchial asthma, and this condition, which has nothing to do with heart disease, is the subject of this book.

Bronchitis is a term that frequently crops up in connection with wheezy breathlessness. The 'itis' has been noted to mean inflammation. So bronchitis is inflammation of the bronchi, the air passages in the lungs. In acute bronchitis the inflammation is caused by an infection, most often a viral infection. Acute bronchitis may occur in people with asthma. When it does so, an attack of asthma may be triggered.

Chronic bronchitis is rather different. The agent causing the inflammation in chronic bronchitis is not an infection; it is atmospheric pollution. For the most part the culprit is that very personal atmospheric pollution caused by cigarette smoking, though industrial pollution can play its part. These forms of pollution work slowly and over a long time; they are chronic. The damage they cause to the air passages results first in phlegm production and chronic bronchitis means simply that: chronic cough with the production of phlegm. Air passages damaged in this way are prone to infection. So, added to the chronic inflammation, there may be episodes of acute bronchitis.

Patients with chronic bronchitis may eventually become short of breath. This is first noticeable on hurrying or climbing stairs. It is an extension of the effects of inflammation on the air passages. The way in which this operates is in some respects similar to that discussed for asthma. But the breathing difficulties of the chronic bronchitic tend to be slowly progressive and not obviously spasmodic. So they do not generally earn the label 'asthma'.

One reason for the inexorably progressive course of the breathing difficulties in this type of patient is the concurrent development of emphysema. Emphysema is a destructive process whereby the lungs gradually lose their resilience. Cigarette smoking is again the chief cause. Patients with emphysema become very short of breath. But this is not asthma.

# 2  How is asthma recognized?

The sensations engendered by a disease are all too familiar to those who suffer from them. To describe those sensations to another is not so easy. Even with pain, one of the most commonly experienced symptoms, it is never certain that the sharpness of a pain will mean quite the same to one person as it does to the next. With breathing difficulties, words seem more than usually inadequate. Perhaps this is because of close links, both biblically and in the popular mind, between breath and life. To take away the breath is to threaten life itself. Such fundamental sensations are not easily described.

Most of us, most of the time have the good fortune to be unaware of our breathing. It is true that exercise can be pushed to the lengths of producing shortness of breath even in the fittest individual. Breathing during exercise is both deeper and more rapid than when resting. There is a certain rawness in the chest—which is due to a drying up of the surface of the air passages and can be relieved by breathing moist air—but the sensation is not unpleasant. Until the point of exhaustion is reached, there is a feeling of satisfaction that the breathing is meeting the demands placed on it by the exercising body. None of this is the case with the asthmatic.

## What it is like to be asthmatic

The presence of bronchial narrowing slows the movement of air into and out of the lungs. There is difficulty both breathing in and breathing out. More effort is required to achieve an adequate flow of air and this increased effort intrudes itself into consciousness. The greater effort produces a sense of difficulty in breathing, which is at the very least unpleasant and can be frightening.

The breathing difficulties of the asthmatic are thus not merely an accentuation of sensations that the healthy amongst us experience during exercise. They are qualitatively different, and demand the use of different descriptive words. Three such words in common use by asthmatics are tightness, congestion, and wheeze. They all refer in some way to that fundamental change in asthma: narrowing of the airways.

The chest tightness experienced by the asthmatic is a direct detection that the airways have narrowed, and that greater effort is required to move air through them. It is an unpleasant sensation that provokes anxiety.

Like many words used to describe symptoms, 'congestion' means one thing to the sufferer another to the doctor. To the medical profession it has a well-defined meaning relating to an unnatural retention of fluid in tissues, and an entrenched tradition connecting this with heart disease. The patient has no such precise ideas in mind when he describes his chest as congested. To him it implies a filling up with phlegm that needs clearing. As such it can be a symptom of asthma. It is also a symptom of several other lung (and heart) conditions.

Wheeze comes from the word Old Norse '*hvaesa*' which meant hiss. It is the sound made by air being forced through narrow airways. Regularly heard through the stethoscope, a wheeze can become obvious to both the asthmatic and to others in a sharp attack of asthma.

Patients may also try to put into words the sensation of distension of the lungs which is consequent on the difficulty in getting air out through narrowed airways. A New Zealand physician who had been a lifelong asthmatic remembered describing this sensation as a child in these words: 'It's just as if your chest had been blown up with a bike pump and then put into an iron clamp'.

## The pattern of asthmatic symptoms

It is not so much the symptoms themselves that enable us to recognize asthma as the circumstances under which they occur. Tightness in the chest, cough, and even wheezing can all occur in other chest diseases. In asthma it is characteristic that they occur in paroxysms. These may be either brief episodes of chest tightness lasting a matter of minutes or more prolonged episodes of wheezing lasting up to an hour or so, which merge into a full-blown attack of asthma.

The asthmatic recognizes that his lungs are sensitive to the weather. Despite warm clothes, the cold winter air 'catches' his chest. There is an immediate tightness, a momentary shortness of breath, but it quickly passes off. The change from a cold outside environment to the warmth of the house might produce a similar brief episode of tightness. There can be sensitivity also to perfume, petrol, wood smoke, cigarettes, and so forth. If exposure is sudden and brief, the tightness is transitory. If the fumes build up slowly, so may the tightness and be all the more bothersome in the end for so doing. The asthmatic is wary too of violent movement of the chest, as in coughing and laughter. Both can set up a paroxysm of wheezing.

These episodes are all examples of the extreme sensitivity of the asthmatic's airways to irritant stimuli. These are not asthmatic attacks—but they are brief episodes lasting perhaps a few minutes of tightness, wheezing, coughing, shortness of breath, that plague the asthmatic's life. It is uncommon for these types of irritation to set off a more prolonged episode of wheezing. This usually requires a stronger stimulus. Perhaps one of the best documented is exercise.

## Exercise-induced asthma

Aretaeus' second century description of asthma begins, 'If from running, gymnastic exercise or any other work, the breathing becomes difficult, it is called asthma'. Shortness of breath during exercise is a common complaint in many types of chest disease. There is, however, something rather different about the effect of exercise on the asthmatic, which almost certainly escaped the notice of Aretaeus. Though the asthmatic does become short of breath during exercise, much more importantly, he becomes even more short of breath after exercise has ended. Instead of being able to relax and 'get his breath back', he finds that a rapidly progressive paroxysm of coughing and wheezing overtakes him. It reaches its peak within a few minutes and he may not recover for half an hour. Virtually no other type of chest disease is associated with symptoms which get worse immediately after exercise, so that this is an extremely valuable guide to diagnosis.

The effects of irritants and of exercise illustrate two aspects of the variability in symptoms that is the hallmark of asthma. There are other patterns. One of the commonest is the waxing and waning in wheeziness which occurs during the course of the day. Many asthmatics will comment on a bothersome tightness in the chest, coughing and wheezing soon after awakening in the morning. With, or even without, the help of morning medicines, the tightness eases in an hour or so, and the rest of the day can be troublefree.

## Nocturnal asthma

An accentuation of this characteristic is for asthma to make itself known during the night. Sir William Osler writes, 'Nocturnal attacks are common. After a few hours sleep, the patient is aroused with a distressing sense of want of breath and a feeling of great oppression in the chest'. There may be an irritating cough which may not even awaken the asthmatic though it often disturbs partner or parents. If awakened, the asthmatic finds breathing is an effort. Muscles around the neck and shoulders are brought into play. There is an obvious and audible wheeze. Sitting up brings some relief and often fitful sleep can follow until with the dawn the attack settles, and, exhausted, a few hours sleep can be snatched. Paroxysms of wheezing like this, repeated night after night, are often associated with a more general wheeziness during the day. This phenomenon of wheeziness in the small hours of the morning or on awakening has become known as the 'morning dip' and is one of the most characteristic features of asthma.

These fluctuations are superimposed on much broader patterns of change that vary considerably from subject to subject. These patterns depend to a great extent on certain specific circumstances which appear to trigger a more prolonged episode of wheezing. They may be seasonal, as with the asthma that accompanies summer hay fever. They may be intermittent as with infections. They may be either brief or more prolonged with emotional stresses. The details of the circumstances which trigger these attacks form the subject matter of later chapters. Most episodes can be aborted or prevented with modern medication but for various reasons, symptoms do sometimes escalate into a full-blown asthma attack. Whatever the cause, there are certain features common to severe attacks which are worthy of mention.

## The asthma attack

Before an attack there may be premonitory symptoms. Aretaeus again: 'The symptoms of its approach are heaviness of the chest, sluggishness to one's accustomed work'. Others describe mood changes, often irritability, which is difficult to rationalize, mixed with depression or apprehension. In a few there is forced gaiety of mood. Before wheezing becomes obvious, coughing is common, not only in attacks at night, but also at other times. It is irritating, rarely productive. Skin irritation with an insatiable urge to scratch is described by some. It especially affects the front of the upper chest. As there will be cause to discuss later, nasal symptoms are commonly associated with asthma. If these have taken the form of a blocked nose, there is a remarkable tendency for the nose to clear early in an asthmatic attack.

At the height of the attack, the dominant feature is the paroxysm of violent wheezing dyspnoea. The sufferer is pale, his facial expression anxious. Beads of sweat stand out on his brow. He feels cold: his skin is clammy. His pulse is rapid and with each breath in, the pulse fades, recovering its force as the breath in is achieved. The soft tissues around the neck and between the ribs are sucked in with the effort of breathing. He sits forward, elbows on knees, or arms resting on the edge of a chair or bed, gasping for breath. Speech is almost impossible save for short broken phrases. He is restless, frightened, and distressed.

Many attacks of asthma settle spontaneously: most today, are aborted by medication, and fortunately few proceed to the extent described by Aretaeus, 'If these symptoms increase, they sometimes produce suffocation after the form of epilepsy'. The easing of an attack is noticed first by the patient himself. The sense of distension is the first to go. It becomes possible for him to breathe out more freely. The wheeze will remain for a while or even increase its loudness as the air flows more easily. Secretions are released; there is both salivation and productive cough. The phlegm is clear or white, sometimes frothy, often sticky and tenacious. It may contain dense white pellets or strands, which occasionally have a branched appearance. They represent casts of mucus which have lodged in the smaller bronchi and have been released as the attack subsides.

After the attack the tension relaxes, the mood elevates. Drink is demanded, some have a great hunger, all want rest.

## Asthmatic coughing and shortness of breath

While the attack is the hallmark of asthma, we must not forget that it can present in other ways such as cough alone or cough with phlegm. These presentations are covered in later chapters of this book. But, in terms of recognizing asthma, it is useful to note that the pattern of timing follows just that described for wheezing. The cough disturbs sleep, comes on after exercise, is a response to breathing in irritants or unaccountably persists long after the cold that went onto the chest should have cleared. Then there is in some asthmatics a more general shortness of breath on exertion. Harping back once more to the eloquent description by Aretaeus, 'During remission, although they may walk erect, they bear traces of the affliction . . . (there is a) difficulty of breathing in running or on a steep road'. This is thus activity-limiting shortness of breath, perhaps associated with wheezing, often not. A patient will say, 'It is not my asthma. I'm just short of breath'. This seems to imply that the anxiety-provoking tightness and distension of the attack are lacking. Due to some permanent but not rapidly variable narrowing of the airways, it is that much more difficult to produce the increased flow of air necessary for activity.

The process of recognizing any disease depends first on obtaining an accurate story. The description just given is the basis on which asthma will be recognized. In an individual much more detail will be required of the circumstances which provoke an attack, in order to identify causes: but more of this anon. Beyond the story, the doctor will want to obtain objective information that he can himself gather which will not rely on the subjective sensations of his patient.

## What can the doctor notice?

There is much in the description just given that is observable. He will note the manner of breathing, the effort put into it, the muscles used, the position adopted. He will note in mild or early stages of an attack the prolonged breathing-out phase. He will note in the more severe attack the increased rate of breathing and the over-inflation of the chest. He will check the pulse for its rate and any variation in its force through the breathing cycle. He will tap the chest to hear the drum-like resonance of lungs distended with air. And he will listen with the stethoscope. Breathing in will be sharp, breathing out prolonged. Wheezing sounds will assail his ears. In very mild asthma they may only be heard after exercise or on forced breathing. In very severe asthma, they may become very soft because so little air is flowing. Sounds of this sort reflect the narrowing of the asthmatic's airways but cannot give an objective measurement of just how narrow they are. For this we need measurements.

## Breathing tests

Direct measurement of the airways in the lung is, of course, impossible in a living subject. It is in any case doubtful if it would be useful for

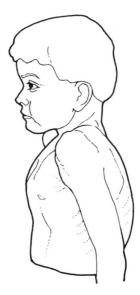

A child with asthma showing the distended chest and raised shoulders.

there are so many of them. In health they vary in diameter from 2 cm to a fraction of a millimetre, and will be widened or narrowed as we breathe in and out. It is in any case not a measurement of size that is required but of function. The airways are used as passages along which air travels to and from the depths of the lungs. In normal airways, air should flow quickly and easily. If the airways are narrowed, as in asthma, flow along them will be impaired.

The principle of the most widely used test of airways function is to see how quickly air can be made to travel along the airways. The lungs are inflated to their maximum extent by taking a big breath in. The breath is held for a moment. The air is then forced out as fast as possible.

The rate at which the air flows out rises very rapidly to a peak value and then declines slowly over the ensuing seconds until all the air has been expelled. Simple measuring devices have been devised which record flow and lock when the peak value has been reached. They are known as peak flow meters and the measurement is called the

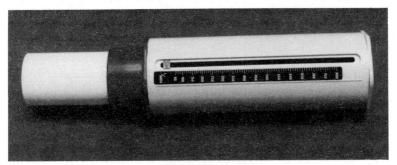

The Wright mini peak flow meter.

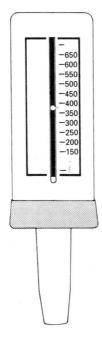

The Vitallograph mini peak flow meter.

**peak expiratory flow rate (PEFR)**. These meters are the commonest devices used to measure lung function in asthma and are prescribable on the NHS.

---

## Using your peak expiratory flow meter

- Set the meter indicator to zero
- Take a full breath in and hold it
- Put your mouth round the mouthpiece and make a good seal with your lips
- Blow out sharply
    do not cough or spit into the meter, just blow out as forcibly as you can
    there is no need to continue blowing out to empty your lungs
- Read off the figure on the scale and make a note of it
- Repeat this procedure twice more
- Record the best of these three readings on your chart or graph

---

The value for peak flow is quoted in litres per minute even though this fast rate is only achieved for a fraction of a second. Normal values lie between 400 and 600 litres per minute. In asthma, values between 200 and 400 are common and in severe attacks peak flow may drop to 100 litres per minute or even lower. The peak flow machine has proved an indispensable tool for measuring the fluctuations in airways' narrowing that are such an important feature of asthma.

There are certain patterns of fluctuation in peak flow that occur in asthma. Several of these will be illustrated in subsequent chapters but one deserves emphasis here. It occurs spontaneously, and reflects the night-time occurrence of asthmatic symptoms described earlier. Even in the healthy amongst us, there is a slight swing in lung function throughout the twenty-four hours. Our airways are narrowest around 4 am, widest open at 4 pm. In the asthmatic, these changes are grossly exaggerated. So if peak flow is measured on awakening, it will be closer to the low values that reflect the narrowing of the airways that occurred at 4 am (hence the term 'morning dip'). A peak flow taken in the late afternoon will be

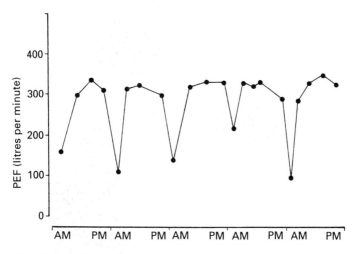

A series of peak flow readings in an asthmatic showing the 'morning dip' due to tightening of the airways during the night.*

Diagrams like this will appear throughout the book. In each instance, the changes in airway calibre will be represented as a change in PEF. Other tests could be, and often are, used but it is simpler to stick with the convention of just using PEF.

much higher. Changes in PEF recorded over several days give a picture just like a saw tooth. Such a pattern is absolutely diagnostic of asthma.

It might well be argued that the speed with which the air can be blown out will depend on the amount of air in the lungs. It does to a degree. This amount can, of course, be measured. The volume of air which can be expelled from the lungs from a point of full inflation to one of maximum deflation is known as the vital capacity (VC). The lungs are not completely empty of air at the end of such a breath. A limit is imposed, chiefly by the bony structure of the rib cage, which clearly cannot be compressed beyond a certain point.

A tall person has a greater vital capacity than a short one. There is an ageing effect. Irrespective of height, the lungs are largest in early adult life. Then there is a steady decline in size with advancing years.

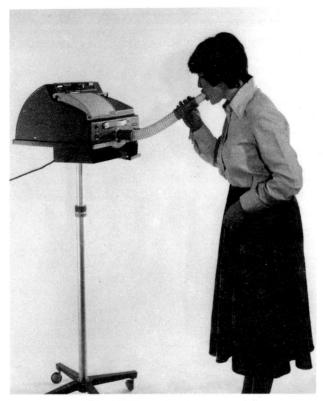

The Vitallograph spirometer.

Finally, men have larger lungs than women of the same height and age. So, in order to obtain some idea of the vital capacity to be expected in a given individual, consideration must be given to height, age, and sex. The same information will allow the peak flow and other tests of breathing capacity to be predicted.

It is possible to measure how much air is coming out of the chest during a forced breath using devices known as **spirometers**. Most spirometers in current use consist of a plastic bellows housed between two hinged metal sheets. Air blown into the spirometer will fill out the bellows and this movement can be registered to give a measure of volume. Portable electronic spirometers are now available but, of course, are more expensive.

### How to use a spirometer

- The spirometer will be set to zero by the doctor or technician
- Take a full breath in and hold it
- Put your mouth round the mouthpiece and make a good seal with your lips
- Blow out forcibly and keep on blowing until your lungs feel quite empty
- You may need to repeat the test several times
- The doctor or technician will analyse the response

All spirometers are geared so that volume can be charted against time. This tracing is known as a spirogram. The slow progress in delivering the air through the asthmatic's narrowed airways now becomes very obvious. The simplest and most useful measurement that indicates speed of delivery relates to the volume delivered after one second. A person with normal airways will deliver 70% or more of his total vital capacity in one second. Narrowed airways will slow this down. So the asthmatic will deliver less than 70% of his vital capacity in one second. It may be 50%: it can be as low as 20%. The actual volume delivered in one second—the forced expiratory volume ($FEV_1$)—will

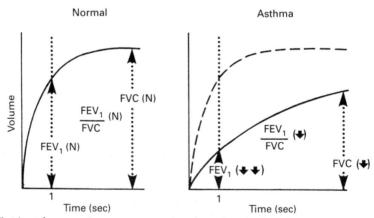

Tracings from a spirometer comparing the reduced values found in an asthma patient with those of a normal person. $FEV_1$: forced expiratory volume; FVC: forced vital capacity; N = normal

depend therefore on the degree of narrowing of the airways. It will also depend, of course, on the size of the vital capacity which in its turn depends on the factors outlined above. This is why it is useful to quote the $FEV_1$ as a percentage of the forced vital capacity (FVC).

Objection can be levelled against tests which depend, as those described so far, on a forced breath out. The very young, who have not yet learned how to control their breathing muscles, will not be able to perform properly. The elderly may find that their powers of control have waned. The very anxious, the mentally disturbed, and the unconscious will not be able to carry out these tests. Co-operation is essential, for to get accurate and meaningful results the breath must be a full one from maximum inspiration to the bottom of expiration and it must be forced out with the greatest possible effort. But despite all this, there is no doubt whatsoever that spirometric and peak flow measurements based on the forced expiratory manoeuvre have contributed enormously to the objective assessment of the asthmatic patient. Above all they are simple to perform, reproducible, and employ cheap and often portable equipment.

Other tests for measuring lung function in asthma exist. They are all less easy to perform and usually employ sophisticated and expensive equipment. They do, however, throw light on the functional disturbances that occur in asthma and so are invaluable for research. It is useful for example to be able to measure the resistance offered by the airways to the flow of air through them during quiet breathing. This may be done using a plethysmograph, a large airtight box with glass sides in which the asthmatic person sits. The plethysmograph can also be used to measure the total size of the lungs including the air left in the lungs after a deep breath out. This reveals that in asthmatics the lungs are blown up. The difficulty in getting air out means that more air remains inside, so the lungs become distended. In mild asthma a modest increase in lung volume may compensate for a slight narrowing of the airways. This is because, as the lungs distend, so do the air passages. In more severe asthma, over-expansion of the lungs is an important cause of distress.

Techniques such as these just described are not routinely employed. They give a clearer picture of the overall disturbance of the functioning of the lungs in asthma, but they are not essential for day-to-day management. For this the peak expiratory flow is entirely adequate.

The recognition of asthma thus depends on a carefully taken story, on observation, and is confirmed by measurement. Both subjective and objective information taken together build up the picture which we recognize as asthma. The circumstances under which asthma occurs provide clues to the cause of asthma. In the next few chapters, some of the mechanisms provoking attacks of asthma will be looked at. First, the fact that asthmatic airways are irritable; then the question of allergy and a description of a variety of other trigger factors including infection, the emotions, and occupation.

# What causes asthma?

# 3  *Irritable airways*

Central to the subject matter of the next few chapters is the question 'What is the cause of asthma?' It is a question to which there is no single answer. Already we have seen that asthma is due to a narrowing of the bronchial airways. This narrowing is caused by mucus, by swelling of the lining of the airways, by bronchial muscle spasm. But what causes the mucus production, the swelling, the spasm?

Some answers can be provided by looking at the circumstances, generally regarded as provoking or triggering an attack of asthma— allergy, infection, and emotional stress. These will all be covered separately in subsequent chapters. Before looking at these specific examples, it is important to recognize that in asthma there appears to be an underlying twitchiness or irritability of the airways. Not only do the airways narrow down in response to the major triggers just mentioned but also to rather less specific insults such as the breathing of cold air or fumes, laughter, and exercise.

It has already been hinted that brief episodes of wheezing like this are likely to be due almost exclusively to spasm of bronchial muscle with little or no contribution from mucus or swelling. So what are the forces controlling the contraction and relaxation of bronchial muscle?

## The autonomic nervous system

Bronchial muscle is involuntary muscle. It cannot, like the muscles of arms or legs, be contracted at will. The nerves which serve involuntary muscle make up what is known as the autonomic nervous system. This part of the nervous system regulates the activity of muscle in the heart, bowel, and bladder, as well as bronchial muscle. It also regulates the calibre of blood vessels, the size of the pupils, and the functioning of many other internal organs.

The autonomic nervous system can be broadly divided into two parts, the sympathetic and the parasympathetic. The sympathetic nerves prepare us for what has been described as 'fight or flight'. The pulse quickens; the blood pressure rises. Blood is diverted from the skin and digestive organs to muscles and brain. The hair stands on end, muscles quiver, pupils widen, and the bronchi dilate. The parasympathetic nervous system, on the other hand, concerns itself with more leisurely digestive and restorative functions. The pulse is slowed and blood is transferred to the digestive organs. Muscles relax, pupils narrow, and the bronchi contract.

## Transmitters

The conveying of information along a nerve and the bringing into activity of muscle are both achieved using a form of electrical energy. There is a small but definite gap between the nerve and the muscle. When it comes to the point of bridging this gap, a chemical messenger, known as a neurotransmitter, takes over.

Different chemicals subserve this function in different parts of the nervous system. For the sympathetic nervous system the transmitter is noradrenaline. For the parasympathetic nervous system it is acetylcholine. When we come to consider the treatment of asthma, clearly one useful aim would be to bring the sympathetic nervous system into play since that results in dilating the bronchi. For the moment our concern is with what causes bronchial muscle to go into a state of contraction. One way in which this could occur would be if the parasympathetic nervous system was brought into action. So let us now consider the evidence that this happens during brief episodes of

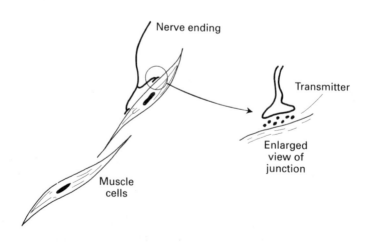

Nerve ending on a muscle fibre.

wheezing and chest tightness, such as occur when the asthmatic inhales fumes, or moves from a warm room out into the cold air.

## Reflexes

Parasympathetic nerve pathways in the lungs are activated by what is known as a reflex. Reflexes are one of the ways in which the human body responds to external stimuli. They are inbuilt, automatic responses and are not consciously instigated. Information received by a sensitive nerve ending is transmitted through central parts of the nervous system and converted into activity that is in some way appropriate to the particular stimulus. There is sometimes a conscious awareness associated with reflex activity. The dropping of a hot plate is a reflex action, but the signal soon gets through that our fingers are burnt. Other reflexes, such as those controlling balance, posture, and movement, operate almost exclusively without our awareness of them.

The most readily understood example of a reflex involving the lung is coughing. A crumb 'goes down the wrong way'. It lands on the surface of the large airways. Here it excites nerve endings. These send messages to the brain which call forth an explosive contraction of the muscles around the chest so that air, and with it the offending crumb, is forcibly expelled from the lungs. This reflex is thus, like dropping the hot plate, a protective mechanism. The nerve fibres leading from surface nerve endings in the airways up to the brain, and those passing back down again to the bronchial muscle, are bound together in a bundle known as the vagus nerve. This nerve is one of the most important parts of the parasympathetic nervous system.

When surface nerve endings further down the airways are excited, the response is not a cough, but a contraction of the muscles in the walls of the airways. So the airways narrow. At first sight this bronchial reflex response again seems to be protective. It attempts to protect the depths of the lung from unwanted particles of dust and irritating fumes, making it more difficult for them to penetrate through narrowed airways. But it also makes it more difficult to breathe them out again. Thinking more carefully it becomes obvious that narrowing the airways is not by any means the most efficient way of coping with unwanted inhaled irritants. Most of all, we have to ask why it happens so much more readily to the asthmatic than to the person with healthy airways?

## Demonstrating airways irritability

A variety of challenges can be used to illustrate that asthmatic airways are excessively irritable. This phenomenon is called hyperresponsiveness. Broadly these challenges can be grouped under three headings:

- physical
- chemical
- allergic (considered fully in the next chapter).

Airways irritability can be studied objectively. Measurements are made of the degree of bronchial narrowing with the person under study resting quietly. The challenge is then given. Further measurements are made repeatedly over subsequent minutes. If the airways are sufficiently sensitive, then the measurements will show an increase in the degree of airways' narrowing. Its extent and duration can be charted. One person can be compared with another by recording the dose of irritant required to cause a predetermined change in the calibre of the airways.

Using a test procedure such as this, known asthmatics can be compared with people who have no asthma. In every instance, and no matter what sort of irritation is used, the airways of asthmatics are more sensitive than normal. In some instances the difference is very striking, of the order of several thousand-fold.

## Physical challenges

One means of providing a physical stimulus to bronchi is the taking into the lungs of a deep full breath. In the asthmatic this will cause a brief but dramatic increase in airways' narrowing. It can be detected within a few seconds of taking the deep breath and is usually gone within a minute. It appears to be a mechanical, reflex bronchial narrowing, and is paralleled in the everyday life of the asthmatic by the wheezing that may follow laughter, or be initiated by coughing. A breath of cold air, a cloud of dust, or a whiff of smoke can all cause an exactly similar effect.

## Chemical challenges

The chemicals chosen are those known to be intimately involved in the chemistry of muscle contraction. They excite very powerful reactions in the airways, and the way in which the bronchi respond to these chemicals has shed considerable light on the nature of bronchial irritability.

The chemical deserving note at this point in the narrative is *acetylcholine*, the chemical transmitter in the vagus nerve which is responsible for the bronchial irritability reflex. When a solution of acetylcholine is made into a vapour and breathed in it causes bronchial muscle to contract. Most tests for assessing this employ a compound closely related to acetylcholine, namely methacholine. Results from inhalation tests with methacholine demonstrate a dramatically increased bronchial irritability in the asthmatic. It requires a great deal of methacholine to persuade normal airways to narrow whereas asthmatics' airways tighten very readily (see figure below). It seems likely that when the methacholine is inhaled, it penetrates through the bronchial wall and so comes into direct contact with bronchial muscles. Not surprisingly, the muscles tighten and so the airways narrow.

A close study of the results of bronchial irritability tests, however,

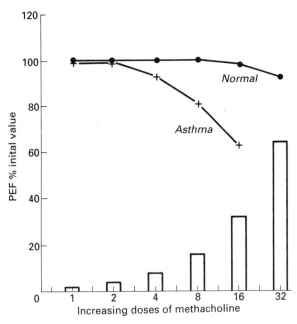

Peak flow responses to increasing doses of metacholine showing how the asthmatic's airways are much more sensitive than normal.

reveals a situation that is not quite as straightforward as might have been hoped. As a symptom, irritability of the airways has been seen to be a hallmark of asthma. But it turns out that there are people with disorders of the airways other than asthma who also show undue irritability to methacholine. Most common amongst these are smokers. Prolonged cigarette smoking renders the bronchi irritable. Bronchial irritability can also be demonstrated in otherwise healthy persons who develop a chance acute bronchitis due to a viral infection, as will be discussed more fully later. So although bronchial irritability is a striking feature of asthma, it is not exclusive to it.

## Exercise-induced asthma

The increased narrowing of the airways which follows the inhalation of irritants is short lived and self-limiting. A more prolonged episode of wheezing is illustrated by exercise-induced asthma. In the previous chapter it was noted that breathlessness which comes on, or gets worse, after exertion has ended, occurs in no other condition. It is understandable therefore that a considerable amount of effort has been expended in trying to understand the mechanism for this type of asthmatic wheezing.

During the course of exercise it is rather difficult to make accurate measurements of airways' calibre, but what information is available suggests that in most people, including asthmatics, the airways widen during exercise. It is what happens after exercise that provides the crucial difference. In the normal person the airways quickly settle back to their previous state. In the asthmatic there is observed a sharp decline in airways' calibre. The airways reach their narrowest about five minutes after the end of exercise, remain at that level for a while, and then gradually widen again. The pre-exercise calibre is usually restored within about an hour but some narrowing can persist for two or three hours. The extent of the change can be considerable. A decrease in airways' calibre by 20% would not be unusual, and the response may be a reduction to over half the initial level.

Exercise can be taken in many forms, and not all appear to be equally capable of producing exercise-induced asthma. Sir John Floyer remarked two centuries ago that for the asthmatic: 'the most agreeable exercise is riding'. Running is certainly the worst. Six to eight minutes free running is recommended when testing for exercise-induced asthma, but many asthmatics will become wheezy

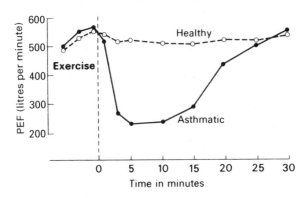

Response of airways to exercise in an asthmatic and a healthy person.

within a shorter time than this. Bicycling will also induce asthma though somewhat less consistently, perhaps because only the legs are used. Kayak paddling, which only uses the arms, is only a mild stimulus. Swimming seems to be the most innocuous of all and so can be recommended to asthmatics. Although both arms and legs are used in swimming, the weight of the body is supported freely by the water. Thus it may be that it is a question of the total amount of energy used that is important in inducing asthma after exercise.

The differences between these forms of exercise are important both to the doctor studying asthma, and, of course, to the patient. In everyday life, the asthmatic will find that the severity of exercise-induced asthma is less with shorter periods of exercise and with light as opposed to heavy exercise. However, quite hard exercise, for example playing football, can be tolerated by the asthmatic, provided it is in brief bursts with some respite in between. Almost all asthmatic children have exercise-induced asthma: it is less common in adults.

## How does exercise induce wheezing?

This remains something of a mystery. Medicines which relax the bronchial muscles, if given before exercise, will prevent the development of wheezing after exercise. So the muscles must be involved. They are probably stimulated to contract by the local release of chemical substances. That some sort of chemical mediator is involved is supported by the fact that a second exercise test carried out within two hours of one test, will produce a much smaller response. This implies that the first test has depleted the stores of mediator, and that it takes time for these to be replenished. A small rise in the level of histamine in the blood has been demonstrated after exercise-induced asthma. So perhaps this is responsible.

*Histamine* is another of the chemical substances that have a special place in asthma. Like acetylcholine, it seems to be involved in the mediation of spontaneous asthmatic episodes; and asthmatics' airways are unduly irritable to histamine as they are to acetylcholine. Inhalation challenge tests can be carried out in asthmatics using histamine in the same way as was described for methacholine. Again, asthmatics are much more sensitive than normal people, but wheezy smokers may be unusually sensitive as well. The release of histamine is especially important in allergic asthma, which will be considered in the next chapter. How exercise causes histamine release is not known.

In recent years exciting advances have been made in our understanding of exercise-induced asthma. Doctors should always pay close attention to the patients' own observations. So when asthmatics commented that their exercise-induced asthma was worse in cold, dry weather than in warm, humid conditions, someone sensibly set out to put this observation to the test. And it was true. The breathing of cold, dry air made exercise-induced asthma worse: and breathing warm, moist air abolished it. At first it could not be decided whether the temperature or the amount of water in the air was important. Now it seems that the water is the culprit. Drying of the air passages is the essential trigger. Cold air is a trigger because it cannot be made to hold water. Indeed the asthmatics' airways seem to be very fussy about the water content of mists breathed into them. Breathing a vapour that is more concentrated in salts than the fluids of the body causes the airways to contract. Equally if asthmatics breathe a pure water mist containing no salts, their airways also show undue irritability. It seems therefore that the very delicate lining of the airways is exquisitely sensitive to the moisture content of the air passing over it, and if the balance of moisture is upset in the asthmatic's lung, wheezing follows.

Before leaving the question of the irritability of the asthmatics' airways, there are two other groups of chemicals that must be mentioned. Their names are somewhat tongue-twisting; the prostaglandins and the leucotrienes. They have attracted a good deal of attention because of the light they throw on the intimate chemical changes that cause asthma. Just as an asthmatics' airways are unduly responsive to histamine and methacholine, so they are very sensitive to prostaglandins and leucotrienes. Tiny amounts of these chemicals when breathed in by asthmatics will produce a brisk asthma attack.

The importance of the *prostaglandins* became recognized when doctors were seeking an explanation for an unusual trigger for asthmatic wheezing—taking aspirin. A very small proportion of asthmatics, perhaps 2–4%, notice that aspirin causes them to wheeze. This is not an allergy to aspirin. None of the tests for allergy, such as those described in the next chapter, are positive. Furthermore it is not a specific reaction. Those sensitive to aspirin are often also sensitive to other substances some of which are chemically quite unrelated to aspirin. These include other painkilling medicines and also tartrazine and benzoic acid—agents used as food additives, in flavouring and colouring.

Several of these substances seem to have one significant property in common. They all suppress the chemical production line that results in the formation of prostaglandins. Prostaglandins are found all over the body. They are of many different types and have many different actions, some beneficial, others probably not. One of the unpleasant features of prostaglandins is that they seem responsible for certain sorts of pain. The reasons for the effectiveness of certain painkillers such as aspirin, may therefore lie in their ability to suppress prostaglandin production.

Prostaglandins when released in the lung affect the airways. Some cause powerful constriction, others relaxation. The balance of these competing prostaglandins is somehow upset in aspirin-sensitive asthmatics. Furthermore when prostaglandin production is suppressed by the aspirin, the body switches its efforts into producing more of the other group of chemicals with an awkward name—the *leucotrienes*. These chemicals come into the story more fully in the next chapter when we take a look at allergic asthma, but undoubtedly they are a powerful cause of asthmatic wheezing in those sensitive to aspirin. The aspirin story is an odd one and not fully explained (there is even an occasional asthmatic who gets relief from aspirin). Despite this, research into prostaglandins has revealed an alternative mechanism for producing asthma, that is neither mediated by nervous pathways, nor is allergic in origin.

The conclusion to be drawn from this rather difficult discussion, which has necessitated excursion into nervous system control and muscle chemistry, is that the airways of the asthmatic possess a rather remarkable irritability. Not only does the inhalation of special chemicals excite a brisk narrowing of the asthmatics' airways, but so does the accidental breathing of dust particles, fumes, and smoke. Even such commonplace disturbances of the even ebb and flow of air in the lungs, as laughter or exercise, can be followed in the asthmatic by embarrassing wheezing and tightness in the chest.

Why it occurs has by no means been discovered. Theories abound, some suggesting an imbalance in the nervous control of the airways, others the presence of unpleasant chemicals produced by inflammation. But whatever the reason airway irritability represents a disturbance of the behaviour of the airways that almost certainly lies at the root of much of the asthmatic's trouble.

# 4  *Pollens, mites, and moulds*

It is widely recognized that asthma may be due to allergy. So what is allergy? Allergy is an unusual sensitivity possessed by some people and not by others. They may be sensitive to particles commonly encountered in the atmosphere, to substances only met in industry, to food eaten, or injections given. The sensitivity may express itself as a rash on the skin, running of the nose, as tummy pain, or, if the lungs are affected, as wheezing. All these sensitivity reactions are in some way unpleasant, certainly unwanted, and even potentially harmful.

The body may react in all these ways at once as a response to certain injections. Indeed, when von Pirquet coined the word 'allergy' at the beginning of this century he was thinking particularly of the body's reaction to the injection of foreign material from other living creatures. Though such injections sometimes produced a violent and unpleasant reaction, at other times the response conferred benefit. Well-known examples of this are vaccination against smallpox and immunization against diphtheria or tetanus. Over the years there has been a tendency to reserve the word 'allergy' for harmful reactions and to use the word 'immunity' for beneficial reactions. But the words are interchangeable and in recent years it has been customary in scientific circles to talk of the study of all these types of reaction as immunology.

In asthma then, the unusual sensitivity or allergy shows itself in the lungs as coughing and wheezing. It is not natural for the lungs to react in this way when foreign material is inhaled. By their very nature the lungs are constantly exposed to foreign particles and fumes present in the air we breathe. The reaction produced in the asthmatic is unpleasant and causes difficulty in breathing. It cannot be regarded as beneficial. So, to further our understanding of how allergy causes asthma we must know a little more about allergy itself.

First, what of the foreign substances which excite sensitivity reactions? These are known as *allergens*. Allergens are nearly always proteins. If they are not, they seem to attach themselves to proteins in the blood before they can set up allergic reactions.

Secondly, to produce an allergic reaction, the body manufactures other proteins which recognize their appropriate allergens. These proteins are termed *antibodies*. The antibody produced against pollen grains is specific for them alone. It will not react with dust particles, diphtheria toxin, or any other foreign material. There are other forms of immunological reaction in which antibodies are not involved, but they can for the moment be disregarded.

Many allergic reactions occur quickly—within a matter of minutes after the antigen has arrived. This is known as immediate allergy. Other allergic reactions only develop after several hours. These are called late allergic reactions.

## Immediate allergy

Immediate allergy is also known as *atopy*. Those who suffer from it are described as atopic. It is the misfortune of a relatively small proportion of the population—about 10 per cent—to have severe atopy, though many others have lesser degrees of atopic sensitivity. Coca, who introduced the term atopy in 1923, used it to describe patients with a variety of conditions which tended to occur together. Asthma was chief among these. Others were: infantile eczema—an irritative inflammation of the skin especially in the creases of the elbows and behind the knees; allergic rhinitis—sneezing, running of the nose, and watering of the eyes suggesting a 'cold' but due to allergy; and urticaria ('hives' or 'nettle rash')—raised red lumps that appear in the skin and itch violently. Coca also added several other conditions to his list, such as migraine and high blood pressure, which today would no longer be accepted as atopic.

The unusual sensitivity which is the hallmark of atopic allergy in these people is reflected in a special reactivity of the skin. However, although those who are atopic in terms of skin reactivity are quite likely to have asthma or other atopic conditions, they do not all have such disorders. Equally, although people with asthma may well be atopic in terms of skin reactivity, by no means all of them are. Because of this, skin reactivity rather than any particular condition, such as asthma or eczema, is now considered a more reliable basis for calling someone atopic.

Atopic skin reactivity is detected using *skin tests*. These are performed with extracts or solutions prepared from allergens found commonly in the environment—fragments of animal hair, pollen grains, household dust, moulds, and so forth. A drop of the fluid is placed on the skin, usually on the forearm. A prick into the surface layers of the skin beneath the drop will allow a minute amount of fluid into the skin. Alternatively the allergen can be dried onto the end of a stillette and this can be pressed into the skin. If the person is sensitive to that allergen a reaction will follow within fifteen minutes. The skin becomes itchy, then red. Finally a small weal, usually about half a centimetre across will form. This positive skin prick test signifies the presence of atopic allergy to that particular allergen.

In certain instances a positive prick test in a person with allergic asthma means that the asthma is directly due to that specific allergen. While this is not always so, it does represent the most straightforward example of allergic asthma. A young girl develops an interest in horses. After a few weeks with her horse she notices a ticklish cough and a tight sensation in the chest. Next she is a little out of breath on running to catch the horse. Then after a vigorous grooming and brushing session she becomes obviously wheezy and distressed. When her skin is tested with horse hair extract there is a positive reaction. The child has asthma. She is atopic. Her asthma is directly triggered by her allergy to horses.

What is happening in her lungs? When the allergen from the horse is first inhaled by the child, it enters the body through the thin surface layer of the airways. There it encounters cells that recognize it as foreign. Antibodies are formed. These are antibodies to the horse hair. They are of a type specifically produced by the atopic person, and called IgE (immunoglobulin, class E). Very little of this antibody is released into the circulation, though modern techniques can detect an excess of IgE in the blood of atopic people. Most of the antibody clings to the surface of rather specialized cells, known as *mast cells*, located in the lining tissues of the bronchi and the skin.

Then the child inhales horse hair particles a second time. In the lungs they meet mast cells coated with specific IgE antibody. Antibody and allergen combine together. This union disrupts the mast cell. It breaks down, and from the interior of the cell granules are released into the surrounding tissues. These granules contain a complex array of chemical substances, which have a wide variety of effects. The first to be released is histamine. It has at least two actions relevant to the production of asthma. First, it causes fluid to leak out of small blood vessels into the loose tissue lying beneath the surface of the airways, so that the tissue swells and the bronchi are narrowed. Secondly, the

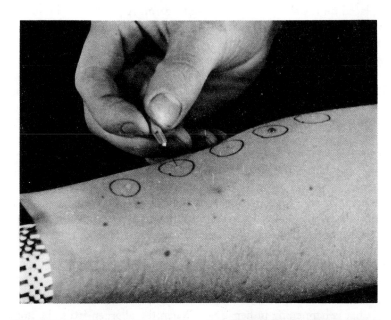

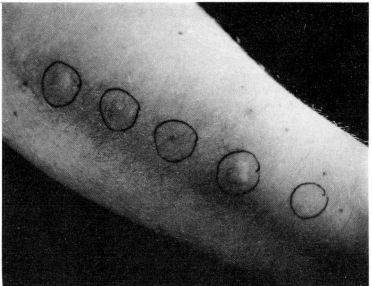

Skin weals produced by skin prick testing with allergens in an atopic person.

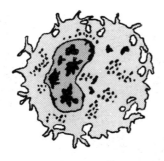

A mast cell.

The interaction between allergens and mast cells in the airways.

histamine makes the muscle in the walls of the airways contract. Once again this narrows the bronchi. Following the release of their histamine, the mast cells manufacture prostaglandins and leucotrienes and release them as well. These substances reinforce the effect of the histamine and sustain the narrowing of the bronchi.

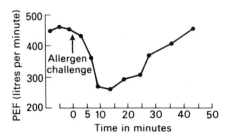

Time course of response of PEF following challenge with an allergen causing an immediate reaction.

With immediate allergy, exposure to allergen will produce wheezing that reaches its peak in 10 to 20 minutes and if there is no further contact with the allergen, it will wane within an hour and will not be detectable after 4 hours.

Asthma in an atopic child sensitive to horses represents one of the simplest examples of allergic asthma. The situation is not always so simple. Indeed the allergies most frequently associated with asthma—to pollens, to mites, and to moulds—each illustrate special features about allergic asthma that repay further study.

## Pollen asthma

Writing over a hundred years ago a middle-aged man recalls a childhood experience. 'I was at the play-work of hay-making with my young companions, surrounded by newly mown grass, when I was suddenly seized with profuse lachrymation, swelling of the eyelids, well-nigh blinding me, and ceaseless sneezing'. His description is of the allergy to grass pollen popularly known as hay fever.

Nasal *hay fever* is common, affecting perhaps one in ten of the population. Much less frequently the hay fever is accompanied by asthma. This is often first heralded by coughing and chest tightness at night during the height of the hay fever season. Then there will be wheezing, day or night, or both. Often a curious reciprocal relationship develops between the chest and the nose. While sneezing and running of the nose are prominent symptoms, the asthma is mild or non-existent. But if the nose becomes blocked, then wheezing builds up.

*Grass pollen asthma* most commonly first makes itself manifest in the first year or two of the hay fever. Both hay fever and purely seasonal grass pollen asthma have a characteristic age of onset. It is unusual for this sort of asthma to start in infancy. It generally begins to appear late in childhood and there is a broad peak of age of onset around puberty which then slowly falls off throughout the teenage period. This contrasts with the distribution of age of onset of asthma in general which has a marked peak in the first few years of life.

With four fifths of the land in England devoted to agriculture, grass pollens from sweet vernal, meadow foxtail, Timothy grass, and a host of others are the usual causes of summer hay fever symptoms. The grasses of the rough pastures of the Scottish highlands and Welsh mountains produce less pollen and on the coast, sea breezes drive the pollens inland. By comparison with his country cousin the town dweller is, to a certain extent, protected against pollen exposure by the forest of stone and concrete that surrounds him.

The grass pollen season covers late spring and early summer. Smaller quantities of pollen are shed before and after this season, extending the period of suffering for unusually sensitive people into early spring

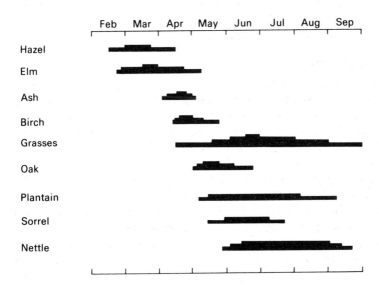

The seasonal distribution of some common pollens in Southern Britain (based on data from Cardiff collected by Drs H. H. Hyde and K. F. Adams, *Acta Allergoligica*, 1960).

or late summer. Symptoms parallel the presence of pollens in the atmosphere. They are greater on a dry, sunny, and windy day and less when rain dampens the spread of the pollen. Most common grasses shed their pollens in the morning, but on a hot day the maximum fall extends into late afternoon.

*Tree and flower pollens* can also cause seasonal nasal symptoms or asthma. Trees flower early, sometimes before their leaves have unfurled. Sneezing and wheezing in early spring may be due to birch pollen: others implicated are elm, hazel, alder, maple, and so forth. Most decorative flowers are not wind pollinated. The scented flowers with their small number of sticky rough pollen grains are insect pollinated. So flower allergy is not common. In North America the commonest summer allergy is to ragweed. Symptoms are commonest in early autumn and have earned the name autumnal catarrh. In Great Britain weed allergy to plantain and sorrel may be admixed with grass pollen allergy. Nettle often causes positive skin prick tests, but it is not at all certain that it is responsible for much sneezing and wheezing.

Pollen grains in the atmosphere can be collected, counted, and identified. Rather different pictures will be given on the same day by collecting devices set up in different localities. It is perhaps unfortunate that the top of a hospital roof in London was chosen to record the pollen count which was broadcast and published each summer day for the information of the British public. Conditions vary so much from place to place that the London figure can be more confusing than helpful. Fortunately, several other centres around the country now publish their own local pollen counts.

With all these summer allergies—whether to tree, grass, or weed pollen—it seems that only a small proportion of those affected by nasal symptoms will develop asthma.

When challenged with histamine or methacholine, people with hay fever alone are just a little more sensitive than normal people. But those with asthma are dramatically more sensitive especially during the pollen season. So the presence of pollen grains in the atmosphere somehow creates the state of increased airways irritability that seems such an essential feature of asthma. But why it does so in some subjects and not in others remains a mystery.

## Dust mite allergy

Asthma occurring with hay fever makes itself obvious by its strictly seasonal occurrence. When asthma is caused by an allergen that is present all the year round, the relation of the asthmatic symptoms to the presence of allergen is much less obvious. Such is the case with household dust. Dust is of course, a complex mixture. It contains fragments of animal and man-made fibres, skin scales, particles of minerals, decorating material, wood, foods, materials such as moulds and pollen blown in from outside, and living creatures, especially insects. The major arthropods are all too familiar to the housewife; she abhors the spider and curses the woodworm. But in the microcosm of household dust are a myriad of tiny mites that escape notice with the naked eye. House dust mites are by far the most important component of household dust as far as asthmatics are concerned.

The commonest house dust mite goes under the stage name of *Dermatophagoides pteronyssinus*. Its life cycle from eggs through to the end of its adult life is up to six months. The mites like a warm, damp environment. Few mites survive long at temperatures less than 5°C. If relative humidity is less than 50% they are quickly desiccated and if above 80% they are suppressed by mould overgrowth. The peak season for live mites to be found is late summer and early autumn. And for food they relish human skin scales. They are not parasitic and only

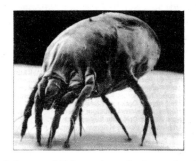

The house dust mite. It is not visible to the naked eye. It takes one hundred end to end to cover an inch.

feed on shed scales. Since each of us sheds about 1 gram of skin debris in 24 hours, there is plenty of nourishment around.

Mites are found wherever man rests for long enough for his skin scales to collect; in the corners of living rooms, on carpets, in cushions and most of all in bedding. There may be 3000 mites in one gram of mattress or pillow dust. They congregate especially in seams and under tapes and buttons. Their life there is almost entirely unmolested by predators. The specific allergens on the mites, and in their faeces as well, can now be identified and their quantity in dust accurately measured.

Early infancy seems to be a critical time for atopic individuals to become sensitized to dust mite allergens. Extent of exposure at this age is an important determinant of dust mite asthma later in childhood.

Household dust has been used to provoke asthma: in the sensitive person it creates an immediate reaction similar to that described above for pollen.

Challenge studies of this sort have an invaluable place in furthering understanding of allergic asthma, but they can only mimic natural exposure to allergen in certain circumstances. The child and her horse are a good example because exposure to the allergen is brief, the wheezing compelling the victim to escape as quickly as possible. Pollen allergy sometimes behaves this way—as when the asthmatic wanders into a meadow in early summer: but more often it is a general tendency to wheeze throughout the pollen season. House dust allergy in its natural form is farthest removed from the simple challenge test. Although dust mites may be concentrated in bedding, they are everywhere. They can be found in the atmosphere at all seasons. The lungs are presented, not with a brief challenge to be followed by an immediate reaction, but by a continuous challenge which gives rise to a persisting state of variable wheeziness. It is important to grasp this point, for it is highly relevant to an understanding of the different patterns of behaviour seen in naturally-occurring asthma.

## Late allergic reactions

While it has not been considered safe to expose asthmatics deliberately to dust or any other allergens for long periods of time, it is feasible to follow some asthmatics for longer than the first hour after allergen challenge. During the second and third hours after the challenge, the chest tightness passes off. But then after about 4 hours in some people, it begins to return. This second phase of asthma reaches its peak at about 10 hours and can last 24 hours or more. It is an altogether more troublesome reaction than the immediate reaction so far described.

What is now happening in the airways? First, they are becoming inflamed and secondly they are becoming irritable, capable of responding excessively to histamine and other chemicals as described in Chapter 3. The word inflammation is now used so commonly in connection with asthma that it needs explaining.

*Inflammation* is a common process affecting our bodies. A sore throat is inflamed: a red swollen joint is inflamed. Food poisoning is inflammation of the bowel: cystitis is inflammation of the bladder. The airways of the lung are most obviously inflamed when we get a cold that goes onto the chest to cause bronchitis. Inflamed tissues become red, swollen, and congested. The blood floods in scavenger cells to fight the infection and clear up the mess left afterwards.

Allergic reactions also cause inflammation but there are several features which make allergic inflammation different. Concentrating on what happens in the airways, we find that in allergic inflammation, there is a more intense swelling of the lining tissues which encroaches on the air passages so narrowing them. Then the inflamed lining produces a sticky mucus that can actually block the airways. The chemical mediators that seem responsible for allergic inflammation include histamine, prostaglandins, and leucotrienes (see previous chapter) which are manufactured by the mast cells. Finally, the scavenger cells that are attracted to airways in allergic inflammation are different from those found in most other sorts of inflammation. The important cell in allergic inflammation is the *eosinophil* (so called because it colours red with the dye eosin). The trouble with the eosinophil is that it would

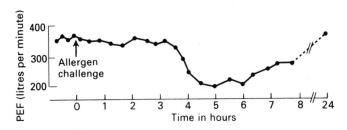

Time course of response of PEf following challenge with an allergen causing a late reaction.

appear not to be very friendly. Rather than clearing up the debris in the inflamed tissues, it seems to break up and itself release complex proteins and chemicals which are harmful instead of healing to the airway tissues.

Eosinophils crowd into the airways during the interval between the early and the late reactions. It is at this time too that the airways become increasingly irritable, increasingly responsive to histamine. And they remain irritable for many days after a single exposure to allergen—or much longer if there is repeated exposure. This is just the sort of situation that occurs in real life, and there is little doubt now that airways inflammation lies at the basis of persistent and chronic asthma.

This part of our adventure into the mechanisms that underlie asthma cannot be left without reference to yet another cell—the *lymphocyte*. Lymphocytes congregate in lymph glands (like the ones that swell up in the neck with infection in the tonsils) but are found throughout the body and in the blood. They play a pivotal role in many immune processes. Lymphocytes become excited or activated when they get involved with an allergic asthmatic reaction. Not only do they encourage more eosinophils to move into the inflamed airways but themselves can release chemicals that make the inflammation worse. Such chemicals are collectively known as cytokines from their ability to make cells ('cyto-') move ('-kine'). Many different cytokines are now being discovered. There is no space for describing them, or their many activities, here, but the term itself needs mention as it increasingly appears in accounts of the cellular mechanisms underlying asthmatic inflammation.

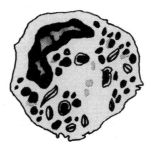

An eosinophil.

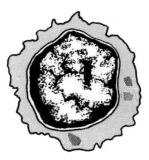

A lymphocyte.

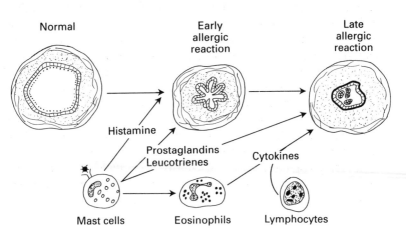

How cells, mediators, and cytokines combine to cause the early and late allergic reactions in the airways.

Lymphocytes are designed to help us cope with foreign invaders by engulfing them, and destroying them through chemical warfare. They can do this with allergens, viruses, and other unwanted material. When this activity takes place in the airways, the end result is the sort of tissue swelling and mucus production that is typical of late asthmatic reactions.

Later chapters will consider forms of asthma which occur in non-atopic individuals. In some of them, lymphocytes appear to play a central role. In others, especially the occupational asthmas (Chapter 8), the situation is unclear or definitely not allergic. Yet in nearly all forms of persistent asthma, inflammation of the airways with eosinophils seems to play a central role.

## Mould allergy

Late allergic reactions can occur with almost any sort of allergic exposure. They are common to all sorts of persistent asthma. Interestingly, late reactions were first recognized in studies on allergy to moulds that date back to 1873. This was the year of the publication of Blackley's book on Catarrhus Aestivus (summer catarrh or hay fever). In it he describes the unpleasant outcome of an accidental challenge resulting from the tipping over of a sample of moulds. He writes, 'After the sneezing had continued a couple of hours, the breathing became very difficult from constriction of the trachea or bronchial tubes. In the course of five to six hours I began to have aching and a sense of weariness over the whole body ... I felt as if passing through an unusually severe attack of influenza'.

Moulds are members of the fungus family. Unlike mushrooms and toadstools they grow on a relatively small scale, producing colonies of growth, often just a few millimetres across, on decaying vegetation and damp walls. Most of the moulds do not have common names, nor are they easy for the layman to identify. *Penicillium*, producing its furry greenish mould on Camembert and Roquefort cheese, is easily recognized. But it is rightly remembered much more as the source of the first antibiotic, penicillin, than as a cause of asthma. Dry rot is also easy enough to recognize. It has a characteristic musty smell and causes a red dust on furniture when its spores are shed in the autumn. These spores, when released into the atmosphere and inhaled, can cause asthma.

Most of the moulds that are important for the asthmatic are less conspicuous. *Cladosporium* and *alternaria* moulds give brownish or grey patches on dead wood or indoor walls. From late summer into autumn very high counts of spores from these moulds can be found in the atmosphere in southern Britain, and many asthmatics who have late summer symptoms seem to be sensitive to them. Spore counts are highest in the warm parts of the day and, like the grass pollen counts, fall in wet weather.

Other moulds are encouraged by the damp and in Britain are most commonly found in the atmosphere in the dank autumn and early winter months. Of these the *Aspergillus* species has been especially singled out for study because of its importance in asthma. *Aspergillus* moulds form grey or black patches on damp walls and very high counts have been found in compost heaps and rotting leaves. In each patch is a branching network of tiny fibres. Sticking out from these are stalks capped by a 'Mop' containing the spores. The name of the mould indeed comes from the Latin, *aspergillum*, which was a mop used to sprinkle holy water in Roman temples!

Aspergillus seems to take an especial pleasure in causing inconvenience to human lungs. For many asthmatics it is one of the potential groups of common environmental allergens like pollens and the house

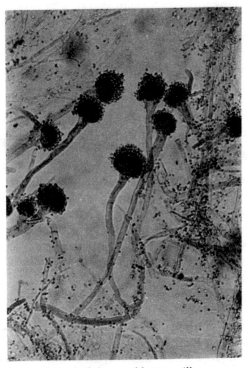

Spores of the mould Aspergillus.

dust mite, that can initiate both the immediate and late types of asthmatic wheezing. But it is also the commonest cause of a rather more vigorous late reaction.

During some late reactions as Blackley described, there is a general upset as well as wheezing, a feeling of malaise, feverishness, and aches and pains of a 'flu-like nature. In fact aspergillus may make itself first known by what appears to be influenza occurring in an established asthmatic. Cough is a prominent feature and very obvious plugs of mucus, perhaps brownish in colour, can be brought up. Aspergillus, unlike other airborne spores, will grow at body temperature and often the mucus plug will contain the mould. Settling in the lungs, these plugs of mucus can block off an airway. No air can then penetrate into that part of the lung: so it temporarily collapses and evidence of this can be seen on the chest radiograph. When the mucus plug is coughed up, the lung re-expands and the chest radiograph clears.

These reactions are also a form of allergy. This time a different class of antibody is manufactured, IgG immunoglobulin. IgG antibodies circulate freely in the blood. This is an advantage since it means that this allergy can be detected using a relatively simple blood test. However, it is not such good news for the asthmatic for it seems to cause much more local damage in the airways. Their walls become weak and tend to balloon out—a condition known as bronchiectasis. Aspergillus allergy is uncommon, but important in what it can teach us about allergic asthma.

Allergy emerges from this discussion then as an important trigger for asthmatic episodes. Immediate allergy may give short-lived attacks in response to allergens such as animal hairs and danders: there may be seasonal wheeziness with pollen asthma: or there may be more persistent asthma in those allergic to house dust. All these allergens are found commonly in the environment, but asthma as a response to them is only observed in specifically atopic people. More prolonged attacks due to late allergy can occur in both atopic and non-atopic people, and are due to a build up of common allergens or to a rather more unusual allergy encountered in special circumstances. The most important of these special circumstances relates to exposure to allergens and other inhaled substances in the work place, and the creation of what is known as occupational asthma. This small but important corner of the asthmatic picture we shall examine in a later chapter.

Some two thirds of asthmatics seem to have at least some of their attacks triggered by allergy and a great deal is now understood about allergic mechanisms. The other major trigger factors, infection and emotional stress, are also important, though less is known of the way in which they cause wheezing. They now have to be considered.

# 5  *Wheezy bronchitis*
••••••••••••••••••••••••••••••••••••••••••••••

Parents frequently report that their children's asthma is triggered by infection. 'When he gets a cold it goes straight to his chest, and he starts wheezing.' Many adults too, especially the more elderly, attribute attacks of asthma to infection.

## What is infection?

Infection has to do with the invasion of the privacy of our bodies by micro-organisms, minute primitive living things. Best known of these are the bacteria and viruses. Each bacterium consists of a single cell protected by a tough outer coat. Viruses are just small fragments of a cell and can only survive and reproduce by residing in another living cell. Micro-organisms are found everywhere. Their food requirements are minimal but their survival is critically dependent on environmental conditions.

Micro-organisms in the atmosphere can settle on the skin but unless they enter the body through a cut or abrasion, they are innocuous. They may be breathed in: a few penetrate into the lungs while most settle in the throat or nose. The surface layers of the nose and throat are quite delicate and frequently abraded. Organisms may reside here without causing trouble, but quite often they gain a foothold, enjoy the conditions, and start to breed. The result is a cold in the nose or a sore throat. The surface lining of the airways is more fragile than that of the throat, but its defences against infection are powerful so that the micro-organisms which penetrate this far, rarely survive for long. If invading micro-organisms do manage to defeat defence mechanisms in the airways, the result is bronchitis or pneumonia. Bronchitis is a street battle. If the battle is carried into the houses, into the depths of the lung, this is pneumonia.

Sore throats, colds in the nose, bronchitis, and pneumonia are all examples of infection. A growth of micro-organisms is the essential feature. Inflammation with swelling, redness, pain, and an out-pouring mucus is the result. Defence mechanisms are mobilized and a battle ensues between the micro-organisms and scavenger cells sent in to fight the infection. The debris from the fray colours the mucus yellow or green. Poisons absorbed from the infected site bring fever, malaise, aching, and listlessness to the rest of the body.

Most often infections of the organs of breathing are due to viruses. The common cold is an example. It is often due to a rhinovirus (literally nose virus), but many other viruses may cause cold symptoms. Unfortunately there is seldom a clearcut pattern of illness which can readily be attributed to a specific virus. Everyone is familiar with the influenza virus. It can cause anything from a mild headache, through sore throats and bronchitis, to a prostrating illness with pneumonia. A viral illness may be complicated by bacterial infection. The disruption caused by the virus creates a fertile field in which an implanted bacterium can happily grow. The prolonged sinus catarrh after a head cold and the persistent coughing up of yellow phlegm after influenza, are both examples of this. Bacterial infection alone is the usual cause of pneumonia.

The majority of episodes of nose and throat infections are nothing more than a bothersome inconvenience. Of those that 'go onto the chest' to cause bronchitis, a majority are, again, minor illnesses. They are characterized by soreness of the chest, cough, and yellow phlegm, but nothing more. It is in a small but important minority that there will also be wheezing.

## Wheezy bronchitis

This concurrence of wheezing with bronchitis is most frequently observed in asthmatics. As many as three out of every four asthmatics regard infection as a definite trigger mechanism for their wheezing. Before unreservedly accepting this view it must be pointed out that it is notoriously difficult to decide on symptoms alone whether an asthmatic episode has been triggered by infection or by allergy. A cold produces sneezing with a runny and blocked nose. So does the nasal allergy that may well accompany allergic asthma. Bronchitis produces coughing with the production of phlegm: so can allergic asthma. Allergic symptoms tend to occur recurrently each time the allergen is encountered. Infections are also sporadic afflictions. An infective bronchitis may give fever and aching limbs and the nasal discharge can become yellow. These last features are not seen with allergy: yet they are hardly firm criteria on which to differentiate infection from allergy.

More objective information is not easy to acquire but is vital in distinguishing these two. The offending micro-organism can be sought in the case of infection. This is frequently a virus. Techniques for catching viruses and persuading them to grow in the laboratory have, in the past, not been too reliable. All this is now changing. In addition antibodies may be sought in the blood. After a recent infection the level of specific antibody to the virus rises temporarily.

So it is now possible to pin-point whether infection or allergy is responsible for a given episode of wheezing. When this is done it emerges unequivocally that infection can, and frequently does, trigger an episode of wheezing in an asthmatic. These viral infections causing wheezy bronchitis are especially common in asthmatic children where they are detectable in 80% or more of acute asthma attacks. Rhinovirus is more likely to be responsible than other viruses; bacteria are almost never responsible.

## Is wheezy bronchitis the same as asthma?

Many children with wheezy bronchitis seldom wheeze at other times. The relationship between recurrent wheezy bronchitis and asthma is a confusing one and one that has been subjected to close scrutiny. The reason for the confusion is partly historical. It was common-place until about forty years ago to call attacks of wheezing in young children, wheezy bronchitis. Doctors thought the term 'asthma' might be frightening and so usually avoided it. And in any case, treatment for asthma was, at that stage, not very advanced. Then two pieces of evidence changed the picture. First a long-term study of children in Australia and secondly a look at the treatment given to wheezy children in Newcastle in the north-east of England.

Primary school children in Melbourne, Australia have been examined at 7 year intervals between the ages of 7 and 28 years. The obvious asthmatics frequently gave a story of hay fever and eczema: skin tests for atopic allergy were almost universally positive. Those who had never wheezed rarely showed these features. But interestingly, those who had just had a few attacks of wheezy bronchitis fell in an intermediate position. They were more likely to show features of allergy than the non-wheezers, though never so frequently as the definite asthmatics. It has also been shown that airways irritability, as judged by exercise testing, can be detected in children who have previously had wheezy bronchitis.

On this evidence wheezy bronchitis in children seems to be a mild form of a condition that in more susceptible children would be called asthma. Good reasons were put forward why these children should be called asthmatic rather than being labelled as wheezy bronchitics. First, it alerts parents and doctors to expect wheeziness under other circumstances such as after exercise or on meeting allergens. And secondly, it means that more appropriate treatment will be given. Antibiotics are not effective for wheezy bronchitis. Treatment for asthma is. Amongst the children with wheezy chests attending school in Newcastle, 95% of those labelled asthmatic were getting the right treatment; but only 50% of those labelled wheezy bronchitics were on the correct medicines.

This lumping together of all children with wheezy episodes under a single heading—asthma—has certainly had a worthwhile outcome in terms of treatment. But as some further surveys are showing, it does hide some important messages. In the south of England, researchers in Southampton managed to observe in some detail nearly 200 children known to have recurrent cough or wheeze. In a twelve month period these children had between three and four episodes of symptoms with a fall in peak flow. Each lasted about four days. Episodes were more frequent in the autumn and winter and were nearly always associated with a viral infection. And what is more, episodes occurred just as often in non-allergic children as they did in allergic children.

These children clearly need long-term scrutiny. Tradition has it that the non-allergic children will grow out of their wheeziness (? asthma) more readily than the allergic ones—but more of this in Chapter 7.

Wheezy bronchitis in adults is rather more difficult to sort out in its relationship to asthma, and this will also be reviewed later in Chapter 7. There is, however, no doubt that at all ages infection can and does trigger an episode of wheezing in the established asthmatic.

## Infection as a cause of asthma

There is now evidence that bronchial infection can itself create conditions which encourage wheezing, conditions that did not exist before the infection had occurred, and indeed might not exist after the infection has finished. It can be shown that previously healthy subjects develop minor degrees of airways narrowing during a simple cold in the head. More significantly, they show increased airways irritability. Whether tested with irritants, with specific chemicals such as methacholine, or with exercise, an undue irritability of the airways often appears during viral bronchitis and for several weeks afterwards.

How frequently does this occur in the population as a whole? It is almost certainly absent or mild in some, and symptomatically significant in only a few. A survey carried out on nearly 400 healthy Norwegians suffering from viral infections found airways narrowing that recovered over 4–6 weeks in more than one in five. Airways irritability was not measured and there was no long-term follow-up. Clinical experience, however, certainly gives the impression that one attack renders the sufferer more likely to further episodes of wheezy bronchitis.

This possibility receives most support from studies in very small children. From about three to six months of age, babies seem unduly susceptible to infection with a virus known as respiratory syncitial virus (RSV). These children develop coughing, wheezing, and distress that is in many ways similar to a severe attack of asthma. If carefully followed up over subsequent years, it seems that about half of these children will have further wheezy attacks, in other words, they become asthmatic.

This outcome seems more likely if the infection occurs very early in life, if the infection is severe, and if there is a family history of allergy. Besides occurring after RSV infection, recurrent wheezing is also seen after rhinovirus infection and occasionally other viruses. Most of these children seem to lose their wheeziness by the age of ten years.

Are attacks of wheezy bronchitis the same as other wheezy episodes, for example those set off by allergy? It is not easy to be sure about this. Certainly there are few asthmatics whose attacks are exclusively triggered by infection, or exclusively by allergy. Both often occur in the same person. However, some patients seem to be able to distinguish bronchitis with wheezing from asthma. It is tempting to dismiss this by saying that they are latching onto clues—such as yellow phlegm in bronchitis—given them by the doctor. But at least one line of evidence suggests that they may be right.

In Chapter 3 on irritable airways, the potential for narrowing the airways—and causing wheeze—through a reflex, was discussed. Viral infections attack the lining of the airways. In doing so they lay bare the nerve endings that give rise to this reflex, making it much more sensitive. We also noted that a chemical called acetylcholine was involved in bringing about this reflex. The effect of acetyl choline can be blocked by anti-cholinergic drugs. The oldest known of these is atropine. In allergic asthma, atropine and its modern equivalents (see Chapter 11) are not very effective. In wheezy bronchitis they can be very beneficial. This suggests that vagal reflexes might be more important in wheezy bronchitis than they are in allergic asthma. So although both wheezy bronchitis and allergic wheezing can occur in the same asthmatic person, they are not necessarily caused through the same mechanism.

## Immunity, infection, and asthma

It is certainly too simplistic to suppose that when infection sets off wheezing it does so solely by vagal reflex irritability. Other possibilities have been explored. One of the more intriguing is that the asthma is an allergic response to the infecting micro-organism.

Part of the body's defence against microbial infection involves creating antibodies. The stimulus for this antibody production comes from protein material in the bacterium or virus just as it does with pollen grains or house dust. Some viruses stimulate a very powerful antibody response. When this happens a subsequent attempt by the virus to invade that host is met with such resounding force that a second infection can rarely take place. This happens with measles, polio, and smallpox viruses. Other viruses are able to attack time after time. Some, like the influenza virus, achieve this by cunningly changing the colour of their spots from year to year. Yet other viruses, like the rhinovirus, seem to exist in so many distinct forms that immunity against one confers no protection against another.

The production of antibodies to invading micro-organisms is largely thought of as a protective mechanism. But could it be damaging? Could an immune reaction between viral or bacterial antigens and the antibody manufactured against them, be harmful? Could this harmful reaction take the form of asthma? There are no definite answers to these questions, but a few interesting pointers have emerged.

First, there is some evidence that, in allergic individuals, specific allergic antibody, IgE (see Chapter 4), is produced in response to viruses (RSV and para-influenza virus). Furthermore, after such an infection, these individuals are more likely to get a damaging late allergic reaction if challenged with their usual allergen, for example, grass pollen. Allergy to bacteria has also been suggested, but not really followed up, since it has become clear that bacterial infection is not important in initiating asthma.

Secondly, viral infections have been shown to increase the frequency of late allergic reactions to common inhaled allergens (see Chapter 4). These normally occur in about one in ten asthmatics. After a viral infection the damaging late allergic response can be seen in eight out of ten asthmatics, and, what is more, this enhancement can last for several weeks.

Then finally, histamine seems to play some part in asthma associated with infection. We saw earlier that histamine is released in the airways in allergic asthma, and causes narrowing of the airways. There is now evidence that viral infections cause excessive histamine to be released, and that some bacteria contain histamine which could leak out into the airways. Histamine release is an important step in encouraging late allergic reactions.

So the second major trigger for attacks of asthma, infection, almost certainly operates in a different way from allergy. Yet it, too, is capable of setting up a state of heightened irritability of the airways. Although this especially happens in existing asthmatics, it can also occur in hitherto healthy individuals. This raises the intriguing possibility that infection can actually initiate asthma in someone who previously did not suffer from it.

Crying and laughter signify a close association between the emotions and breathing. Excitement and horror can cause us to catch our breath. Can the emotions cause wheezing? There is a long tradition that says they can. Hippocrates warned the asthmatic to guard against anger. Sir William Osler echoed this belief nineteen centuries later with the comment 'fright or violent emotion of any sort may bring on a paroxysm', and in his textbook of medicine stated, 'All writers agree that there is, in a majority of cases of bronchial asthma, a strong neurotic element'.

There was a flowering in the 1920s of interest in the ways in which psychological forces could induce and perpetuate bodily illness. Yet in the past three decades the study of allergic mechanisms in asthma has all but eclipsed any consideration of emotional influences.

## The lady and the rose

John Mackenzie, an ear, nose, and throat surgeon of Baltimore, writing in 1885 described a woman with summer seasonal hay fever and asthma, ascribed, as it often was, to the scent of roses, 'Mrs. A., thirty two years of age, in excellent circumstances, surrounded by all the comforts of life; very stout, well nourished, but physically weak . . .'. Her asthma had begun at the age of 12 years, was summer seasonal and associated with typical itching of the nose and paroxysms of sneezing. Attacks of wheezing could be provoked by innumerable circumstances which included the odour of hay and roses. Mackenzie writes on: 'Decidedly sceptical as to the power of pollen to produce a paroxysm in her particular case. I practised the following deception upon her . . . I obtained an artificial rose of such exquisite workmanship that it presented a perfect counterfeit of the original'. During an interview 'I produced the artificial rose . . . and, sitting before her, held it in my hand, at the same time continuing the conversation. In the course of a minute she said she felt that she must sneeze . . . The nasal passages became suddenly obstructed . . . In a few minutes the feeling of oppression in the chest began with slight embarrassment of respiration'. It caused her great amazement to learn that the rose was artificial but the effect was wholly beneficial. A few days later she reported that she had buried her nostrils in a large fragrant specimen of the genuine article without the slightest ill effect.

## Conditioning

This story is probably an example of conditioning. Allergy had not been clearly defined in 1885. Yet it must be supposed that the lady's asthma had been initiated by allergy to pollen. On this background a psychological mechanism operated. Her fear of developing wheezing on contact with roses was sufficient to cause her in fact to wheeze even though the rose was artificial.

Attempts have been made to reproduce this under more carefully controlled conditions. Two asthmatic women known to be sensitive to pollen were repeatedly tested with inhalations of pollen extract and an inert solution containing no pollen. At first they regularly developed wheeze with the pollen but were uninfluenced by the inert solution. They were not told which solution to expect. After several days of testing, they began to react to the inert solution as well as to the pollen. Next, wheezing was detectable when air alone was blown at them with no solution at all. Finally, the mere act of putting on the mouthpiece to start the test was sufficient to set off a reaction.

It is unfortunate that the assessment of wheezing in these studies depended on spirometric tests which can be influenced by motivation. One wonders what was so special about these two asthmatics and in how many others such an effect could have been produced. The experiments lack, too, some of the sophistication put into conditioning studies now. Yet if nothing else, these two women did reveal the power suggestion has on the airways.

## Suggestion

Some of the most scientifically controlled studies of the influence of suggestion on asthma were carried out in the late 1960s by Luparello and his colleagues. Forty asthmatics allowed themselves to be subjected to a number of studies in which their lung function was assessed by techniques not dependent on cooperation or motivation. Measurements were made before and for four hours after the inhalation of an aerosol, which was simply a dilute solution of salt. The patients were told, however, that it was an allergen to which they knew they were sensitive. In almost half these asthmatics there was evidence of increased narrowing of the airways and in a quarter there was an obvious attack of asthma. In those who wheezed, a second inhalation of the same salt aerosol was given. This time they were told it was a treatment which would relax their airways. It did. Attempts to repeat these studies subsequently have not always been successful. Yet when they have, it has been clearly shown that medicines which counteract the activity of the parasympathetic nervous system (see p. 47–48) will prevent suggestion from causing narrowing of the airways.

Those individuals who respond to suggestion are also often those who can be readily hypnotized. The use of hypnosis in the treatment of asthma is the logical outcome of these observations and the degree to which it has been successful we will judge later. An effect attributable to suggestion alone is an important facet to the assessment of new drug therapies in asthma. The active drug must always be checked against an inert 'placebo' preparation. In children, for example, some protection against wheezing after exercise can be obtained in 40% by the use of a placebo.

## Environmental stress

The production of asthma by images of potentially allergic stimuli is one facet to the interaction between psychological forces and asthma. Another is the direct provocation of wheezing by psychological stress. Careful questioning of unselected asthmatics reveals that they often feel that their emotional state influences their asthma. Dr Storr described in his introduction how, in him, undue stress provoked asthma. Many patients would echo his experience. The range of emotions implicated is wide—anger, anxiety, depression, guilt, even pleasurable excitement and joy. The triggering of attacks of wheezing by emotional stress can be recorded in up to 70% of asthmatics; but it is very rarely the only trigger. Indeed, it is perhaps the interaction between emotional and non-emotional factors that is of most interest.

## The dishonest coachman

This is revealed in an anecdote told by Trousseau, a notable nineteenth century French physician, about himself. He was an asthmatic. His worst attack of asthma occurred in a grain loft. The air was dusty but on this occasion there was an emotional charge in the atmosphere. Trousseau suspected his coachman of dishonesty in measuring the oats, and had decided on this occasion to supervise the operation. 'I had a hundred times been exposed to an atmosphere of dust considerably thicker . . . This time it acted on me whilst I was in a peculiar state. My nervous system was shaken from the influence of mental emotion caused by the idea of a theft, however trifling, committed by one of my servants'.

This type of interaction between emotional and allergic stimuli is potentially more relevant to the everyday life of the asthmatic. It has been studied objectively. A small dose of pollen extract was released into the atmosphere unbeknown to the patient and insufficient to cause any wheezing. An interviewer then discussed various aspects of that patient's asthma with him. If the discussion touched on unpleasant circumstances associated with his asthma, then wheezing was provoked; if these topics were avoided there was no wheezing.

Although some anomalies are encountered in relating emotional stress to wheezing—such as why stress can both heighten and relieve wheezing—there is no difficulty in proposing ways in which psychological events might influence the airways. Higher centres in the brain can cause the airways to contract through the parasympathetic nervous system. Indeed, medicines which antagonize parasympathetic nerve activity partly reduce the adverse effects of suggestion on the airways. Conversely, stress activates the adrenal glands to secrete hormones which can relax bronchial muscle.

There is now mounting evidence that psychological stress can influence the immune system. Defence against the common cold is less good in individuals subject to stress. The pattern of release of chemicals in inflamed airways may be adversely affected by stress, and this could be a mechanism through which stress exacerbates asthma.

## The empty goldfish bowl

A further case history will serve to underline points already made in relation to suggestion and conditioning, and introduce another facet into this narrative. An asthmatic woman known to be allergic to pollens and house dust believed herself to be allergic to goldfish. This seemed strange since there was no way in which the goldfish could give off any allergens that could be inhaled. Under circumstances where lung function tests could be carried out, she was shown a live goldfish in a bowl. She became wheezy. On a second occasion she was shown a toy goldfish in a bowl. Despite the fact that she realized it was ridiculous, she again became wheezy. Finally she became wheezy when shown an empty goldfish bowl.

During the course of these tests she had a dream. In her dream she saw a huge goldfish bowl. On a shelf high above it were her books. She wanted to read why goldfishes cause asthma. She climbed on a chair and reached for the book, but it was too high. She lost her balance and fell into the goldfish bowl. The fishes swam around. She gasped for breath. Her neck became caught in a strand of water weed. Suddenly she was awake, wheezing, and fighting for breath.

This patient also described how, when she was a child, her mother had thrown away her goldfish, which she had loved very much and had saved her pocket money to buy. The memories became all too real, when in an attempt to stop her wheezing in the final study the experimenter smashed the goldfish bowl. The wheezing intensified. 'That is exactly what my mother did', she exclaimed; 'she threw the bowl into the dustbin'.

## Parents and children

The implication from this account is that tension between the asthmatic and her mother was in some way responsible for the child's asthma. Various aspects of the parent/child relationship have been thought to be significant perpetuating factors in childhood asthma. The removal of an asthmatic child from home to hospital is often accompanied by immediate and dramatic improvement. The change seems disproportionate to the effect that might be expected for removal from environmental allergens. Cats, dogs, and household dust may be important triggers but there is a suggestion that they act on a background of psychological stress.

## Trials of separation in Holland and North America

When asthmatic Dutch children were sent to Switzerland during World War II they were certainly being removed from the influence of the house dust mite. This creature survives poorly in the dry heights of the Alps. The children improved: and they did rather better than local Swiss asthmatic children. After the war, a residential school for asthmatics was set up in Holland itself. The Dutch children showed just as much improvement in their asthma when in the Dutch school as they did in Switzerland. The Dutch residential school had as many mites as the children's own homes. The common feature between the residential schools was not removal from household allergens, but the separation of the children from their parents.

In Denver, Colorado, in the USA, a residential home has been run since the 1930s for children with chronic severe asthma. They remain there from 1 to 3 years. As few as one in 20 fail to benefit from their stay. On returning to their own homes, half of these children require no treatment, and the remainder manage well on reduced treatment. That the separation of the children from their parents is critical in this exercise is made clear from a reversal of the usual separation procedure. Instead of removing the child to a residential home, the parents were moved into a hotel and appropriate provisions made for the children in their own homes. For those children in whom family tensions were felt to be important, the results were beneficial.

The root of the tension in these children often lies in the over-protective attitude of their parents. It is distressing to see a child with acute asthma. It is natural for parents to do all they can to protect their children from environmental allergens, from 'catching cold', from the mockery of school fellows: but it can be carried too far. One of the benefits that follow removing a child to hospital may be the stimulus it gives to the child to become independent from an understandable but stifling attitude by parents.

Other features of living at home which seem to be associated with recurrent severe asthma are quite the reverse and stem from deprivation. Neglect caused by poverty and overcrowding, marital disharmony, parental separation, the death of a parent, are all mentioned. None are specific causes for asthma. But they are all potentially serious for the child with irritable asthmatic airways.

## How important is stress in asthma?

These observations leave little doubt than in some childhood asthmatics, there is a sufficient background of tension in the home to make this a significant factor in the persistence of the child's asthma. But how often does this happen? The Denver physician states, 'I selected only the sickest for admission in the home'. There is no satisfactory information on which to base a reliable estimate. About a quarter of the children attending an asthma clinic at a London teaching hospital were described as having severe perennial asthma. These would be the type of patients from whom the Denver children were selected. But since only about one in five of childhood asthmatics attends a hospital clinic, the number who might be suffering in this way is likely to be well under 5%.

Set against this small minority of childhood asthmatics is the vast majority in whom emotional tensions play a minor or insignificant role. The excitement of parties or holidays may bubble over into wheezing and not infrequently there is an element of manipulation perhaps, for example, in relation to examinations. Yet in general the attitude of children is more one of domination over, rather than domination by, their asthma.

## An asthmatic personality?

It has been suggested that if asthma can be influenced by psychological events, asthmatics ought to have a readily identifiable personality. Analyses of the personality traits of asthmatics are legion. Asthmatics have been described as irritable, easily aroused to anger, whining, complaining. They have been categorized as obsessional neurotics. They have been seen as lacking self-confidence and frequently depressed.

Defects exist in many of the studies making it difficult to interpret the findings. Inappropriate questions have been asked or inadequate control studies carried out. Overall, there seems to be no clear cut evidence that there is a specific asthmatic personality. Perhaps it is fair to comment on some of the better studies to illustrate the extremes of opinion.

Those who most strongly support the concept of a specific asthmatic personality are the psychoanalysts. They start with the asthmatic's frequently voiced opinions of himself: 'I don't show my feelings easily': 'I bottle things up'. The free expression of emotion brings relief. To inhibit emotional expression invites tension. The suggestion is that in the asthmatic, the tension is reflected in the lungs. This conversion of emotional tensions into a bodily disorder makes the conflict more socially acceptable. Even today the sight of an asthmatic wheezing engenders more pity than does overt neurotic disturbance. The suppressed emotion is generally not consciously appreciated. If it can be revealed and the tension broken, the asthma may clear. This has been described. A young woman, asthmatic since childhood, recalled under psychoanalysis a scene from her childhood in which someone had been strangled. Her fear had been suppressed and, with it, her memory of the event, but she became asthmatic. Treatment enabled her to resolve her fears and her asthma disappeared.

## Suppressed crying

Children occasionally seem to be able to manipulate their asthma consciously. 'I think myself into an attack'. Indeed whether consciously recognized or not, it is in childhood emotional conflicts that the psychoanalysts find most support for their theories. The most specifically enunciated conflict related to asthma is that it is a form of 'suppressed crying'. Here we have the disturbed parent/child relationship again. The child loves his mother intensely yet feels her rejecting him. Crying would alienate the mother further, but its conversion into asthmatic wheezing calls forth her pity and love.

Anecdotal support is easy to find amongst the famous. Marcel Proust was pathologically attached to his beloved 'Mamma'. Yet he frequently quarrelled with her, and suffered many bouts of wheezing as a result. In his youth, Theodore Roosevelt was asthmatic and clearly very close to his mother. When aged eleven he wrote, 'I was very sick last night and Mamma was so very kind telling me storys (sic) and rubbing me with her delicate fingers'. Throwing off his dependence in his teens, Roosevelt's asthma ceased to bother him seriously.

## Psychological and physical disability

This firm confidence in a specific type of emotional conflict being responsible for asthma is not widely shared. It has been pointed out that many surveys have suggested that asthmatics are unduly neurotic, anxiety-prone, and obsessional. Two reservations make the validity of these comments suspect. The first is illustrated by a comparative study from Edinburgh. In this, the asthmatics were compared with a control population which included those who were in robust mental health and those who were frankly neurotic. The degree of neuroticism elicited amongst the asthmatics was halfway between the two extremes: and so was the average of the control population as a whole. In other words, asthmatics are a bit neurotic. But so are we all!

The second reservation arises from studies in which asthmatics have been compared with those having other types of physical handicap. The asthmatics appeared no more anxious, nor neurotically disturbed in any specific way than others with a physical disability. This raises the classic hen and egg argument. Did the anxious personality precede the development of the asthma and perhaps in some way contribute towards it? Or did it arise as a result of constant fear of another attack and anxiety over school or work prospects?

There can be no specific answer to these questions nor any definitive assessment of the role of psychogenic factors in asthma. None would argue with the view that anxiety and stress may trigger an attack in an established asthmatic. Most physicians know of patients in whom psychogenic factors have seemed to be responsible for the initiation of a spell of asthma, or have contributed to the perpetuation of asthma once established. But few would regard this as common and would not concur with the view that there is a specific personality type universally encountered in asthmatic patients.

Finally it must be remembered that breathlessness itself carries psychological overtones. The difficulty in drawing breath whether experienced or anticipated can itself engender a state of tension that will intensify any distress directly attributed to the airways narrowing.

# Environment and heredity

# 7 Age and inheritance

Previous chapters have given a description of airways irritability and of the major trigger factors for attacks of asthma—allergy, infection, and emotion—which has created a picture of asthma in individuals. These miniature portraits need to be collected together on a broader canvas. The scene that emerges has certain themes. These relate to the temporal pattern of asthmatic symptoms, the balance of trigger factors, and the changing face asthma presents at different ages.

## Patterns of asthma

### Intermittent and continuous asthma

Asthma is a disorder of great variability, sometimes troublesome, at others unnoticed: sometimes mild, at others serious. The asthmatic's irritable airways may respond to fumes, to laughter, to exercise, with a brief spasm of wheezing or coughing that passes off almost as readily as it came. Between such episodes, though the potential for becoming wheezy remains, the airways are clear. The asthmatic sensitive to cats or to horse hair, or pollen will have symptoms when these allergens are in the air: but at other times his airways, unmolested, cause him no distress. An attack of wheezy bronchitis may carry in its train several days, or even weeks, of shortness of breath, wheeze, and productive cough but, with treatment, it all recovers and once more the asthmatic breathes freely. Stress or anxiety will heighten wheeziness for a while but with the easing of tension or the acceptance of disappointment, the airways relax again. All these are commonplace facets of asthma as it is experienced by the majority of asthmatics. Their asthma is intermittent: between attacks they are completely free of symptoms.

A pattern of intermittent attacks is not only the common way that asthma presents, it is the least serious. At all ages those with intermittent attacks are most likely to remain in good health, to be minimally bothered by asthma, or to lose their asthma altogether.

Intermittent asthma may be contrasted with the pattern of asthma in those who have some degree of shortness of breath between attacks.

This pattern of asthma is given various labels. Some call it 'continuous', others 'persistent' asthma. Yet others would use the term chronic asthma to describe symptoms that persist over many weeks, months, or even years.

Continuous asthma contrasts with intermittent asthma in several respects. Not least amongst these is the poorer outlook with which it is associated. Asthmatics with continuous symptoms are only half as likely to lose their asthma as those with intermittent symptoms. The drawing of this contrast between intermittent and continuous asthmatic symptoms illustrates one broad pattern that can be used to divide up asthmatic patients. A second feature of this division relates to age of onset. It emerges that four out of every five of those with intermittent asthma begin to wheeze before the age of 16 compared with just half of those with continuous asthma.

## Extrinsic and intrinsic asthma

Contrasting intermittent with continuous asthma is a division by clinical pattern. Others have used a division based on 'cause'. The best-known is that of Rackemann who described his asthmatic patients as either having 'extrinsic' or 'intrinsic' asthma. In extrinsic asthma 'the attacks are due to contact with foreign substances in the environment outside the body': this is thus virtually synonymous with asthma due to allergy. With intrinsic asthma the cause was believed to lie somehow within the patient. It was, at least initially, thought to be a specific reactivity to infection. In such patients skin prick tests for atopic allergy were negative, whereas they were positive in the extrinsic group. The contrast drawn between extrinsic and intrinsic asthma does somewhat follow the clinical pattern of intermittent versus continuous asthma, but not closely. Extrinsic asthma is often intermittent, but quite often allergic factors are found in those with continuous symptoms. The age feature crops up again: Rackemann writes: 'When asthma begins before age thirty, the cause is allergy unless proved otherwise: but when asthma begins after age forty, the cause is not allergy unless proved otherwise'. Such broad generalizations, although subject to many individual exceptions, help to create an overall picture of asthma.

The term intrinsic asthma has been subjected to many nuances of meaning since its introduction. It has been used when no specific cause could be found for the asthma. It has been regarded as synonymous with infection causing asthma. In the absence of external environmental allergens, infection is certainly a frequent trigger but even so it is not necessarily the underlying cause of the asthma. Intrinsic has been applied to the condition of patients with continuous asthma where a whole variety of factors may precipitate wheezing.

To draw a clear distinction between extrinsic and intrinsic, allergic and non-allergic asthma is almost certainly too simplistic. Though allergy is a common trigger, it is rarely the only cause of wheezing in an individual. Infections are seldom singled out by patients as the sole occasions on which they wheeze. It is likewise with emotional stress. All three can at some time be a trigger for asthma in an individual and one trigger is seldom the sole cause of asthma. It is more often a constellation of circumstances which sets off asthmatic symptoms.

## Irritable airways as the basis for asthma

Asthma emerges from any analysis such as this, not as a specific condition with a specific cause, but rather as a disturbance of the behaviour of the airways. They are irritable. It is not a feature of healthy airways to tighten up when there is a chance breathing in of cold air. A few pollen grains or some specks of household dust are harmless except to the sensitive asthmatic. Bronchitis is a common ailment: it is not normally accompanied by wheezing except in the asthmatic. Emotional stress is an accepted hazard of life: only in the asthmatic may it cause the airways to narrow. The environmental irritants, allergens, infections, and stresses which assail the asthmatic differ in no way from those the rest of us experience. It is in their impact on the way in which the airways function that the difference lies. Indeed it is the very irritability of the airways that would seem to be the underlying defect.

It has now clearly been shown that an attack of asthma can heighten airway responsiveness whether it is triggered by allergy or by infection. What is not yet certain is whether some people are predisposed to develop irritable airways, nor how often it evolves entirely due to encounters with allergies or infections in the environment. What has been discovered we shall examine at the end of this chapter.

Hints have already been given that asthma varies in the way it presents and behaves at different ages. It starts most commonly in childhood and it is here we should begin to look at asthma through the ages.

# Childhood asthma

Asthma is common in childhood. In England and Wales there are at least half a million children with diagnosed asthma and a similar number who wheeze sufficiently often to deserve being so diagnosed. It is indeed the commonest chronic disease of childhood. Despite this, for most children, their asthma is not troublesome, and in only a few can it be described as severe.

For the most part asthma in children presents a pattern of episodic wheezing. Infection and exercise are the commonest triggers for childhood asthma attacks. Three-quarters of all asthmatic children suffer no more than infrequent mild attacks of wheezing with long free intervals between them. They cause no real disturbance to daily life and are easily treated with simple remedies. In schoolchildren from Melbourne, Australia, it was found that over half the asthmatic children had a total of less than ten attacks of asthma by the age of ten years.

Despite it being a common and relatively benign disorder, there is much about childhood asthma that is fascinating and unexplained. One of the most remarkable is the observation that in early childhood boys are more likely to have asthma than girls, the margin being of the order of two, even three, to one. This excess evens itself out gradually and is lost by the teenage years.

The reasons why asthma starts in young children are complex. As we shall see in more detail later, those children who inherit a tendency to develop allergies are more likely to become asthmatic than those who do not. At present there is no known way of avoiding this. On the other hand, there is a clear message for prevention in the observation that the children of mothers who smoke more than ten cigarettes a day are twice as likely to become asthmatic as the children of non-smoking mothers.

## Early childhood

Asthma in children presents special features at different ages. Starting with the youngest, we have the 'fat, happy wheezers' of the first year of life. Doctors are reluctant to diagnose asthma in infancy, yet wheeziness in babies is not uncommon. The usual story is of a dramatic attack of distressing cough and wheeze following what appears to be a cold or sore throat. After two or three days the intense symptoms settle and recovery is usually complete within a week. During the attack little, if any, benefit seems to come from the usual therapies that help asthmatic children. Up to a half of these wheezy babies may have further attacks, and for some years through childhood they have irritable airways. Fortunately, very few appear to become truly asthmatic children. It seems that unless these, presumably viral, infections by chance occur in a child predisposed to develop asthma, no lasting harm follows such attacks. An exception already mentioned is the recognized tendency of asthma to follow infection with the particular virus known as RSV.

Then there is the quite common presentation of asthma especially in pre-school children as coughing alone without any wheezing being obvious. Because of this, thoughts will not immediately turn to asthma, but a careful analysis of the circumstances under which the coughing occurs will reveal that it follows the same pattern as that described for wheezing. Thus the coughing will be most obvious during the night, on awakening in the morning, and after exercise. There is an unfortunate tendency for these children to be regarded as 'bronchitic' and to be treated with antibiotics. As we discussed in the chapter on infection, this is the wrong approach. They are asthmatic and should be treated as such.

Asthma may develop quite gradually on top of a story of essentially nasal symptoms. These children have what seems to be recurrent colds with a running and then a blocked nose. They are dubbed 'catarrhal'. Wheezing appears without an obvious trigger, perhaps first at night, or after exertion. The asthma is not severe, just intermittently bothersome. There is a no story of bronchitis and there are no other features pointing to infection.

Exercise-induced asthma (see Chapter 3) is almost universal amongst children. Perhaps because their natural exuberance makes them more active, they will complain more about exercise bringing on cough and wheeze than do more sedentary adults. Likewise, children may bitterly complain that other physical triggers such as laughter or crying also set off their asthma.

## Allergy and childhood asthma

It is tempting to suppose that many of the features of childhood asthma are due to allergy, but an attempt to tie up symptoms with exposure to some agent likely to cause allergy, generally fails. Indeed, asthma in children which is unequivocally and solely allergically precipitated is quite uncommon. There are individual children who only get asthma after contact with a horse, a cat, or a dog: but these are a minority. Asthma during the pollen season is a somewhat separate problem occurring in rather older children and will be considered later.

Though asthma in children may not often be due exclusively to allergy, yet a close and fundamental relationship exists between atopic allergy and childhood asthma. There is a striking concurrence of infantile eczema and rhinitis with asthma in certain young children. The eczema comes on in the first year of life; perhaps it is only in the creases of the elbows and behind the knees, or the wrists, hands, trunk, and face may be affected as well. Persistent 'colds' afflict the child's nose and by the age of two years he has usually had his first attack of wheezing. The asthma is well established by the school years. It is these children that make up the majority of those who go on to have persistent symptoms. Indeed, two-thirds of children with frequent persistent asthma have, or have had, eczema: and over 90% of them show positive skin tests of the atopic type. Some eczematous, asthmatic children have a food allergy, often to dairy products, and can be helped by exclusion diets. However, sensitivities to food or drink, though much discussed, are seldom the sole cause of childhood asthma.

The more seriously affected children are then more likely to be highly allergic. Their asthma often begins early in life and, unlike the fat happy wheezers, these children are frequently made miserable by their asthma. It does not settle properly between attacks, and some will have persistent symptoms by the age of five years or so. Sleepless nights due to coughing and wheezing leave the child weak and breathless in the day. Often much time is lost from school. Their chests become overinflated and bear the hallmarks of the constant fight for breath. Fortunately the numbers of such children are small and most gain relief from modern therapy. They seldom, however, completely lose their wheeze later in life.

Atopic allergy and asthma march closer together in childhood than at any other age. Despite this, allergy alone cannot explain all the vagaries of the behaviour of asthma in children. What allergy can induce wheezing after laughter or exercise? Are the emotions allergic? And what of the many children who show positive skin tests but who have no asthma? For every atopic child with asthma, there are two who are atopic but do not have asthma. The atopic state can clearly exist without asthma. Is the reverse true? Not very often in children. Only 7% of the Melbourne children with severe asthma never had positive skin prick tests at any stage during 14 years of observation. However, about half of those with mild or infrequent asthma were always skin test negative. It looks as though in most instances the irritability factor, best exemplified by exercise-induced asthma, must interact with atopic allergy, best exemplified by positive skin tests, before asthma can develop. Despite this a very few asthmatic children do not have exercise-induced asthma and a very few do not have positive skin tests.

Wheezing in children is nearly always then due to either infection or allergy or both, creating an asthmatic state. There are alternative explanations—such as a particle of food or other foreign body 'going down the wrong way' or acid from the stomach coming back upwards and affecting the lungs—but these are rare.

## Asthma in the school years

Two issues have surfaced in recent years concerning ways in which asthma affects the everyday life of children, and these deserve attention. The first is the question of under-diagnosis: the second concerns how asthmatic children fare at school. Under-diagnosis was first brought to light in a survey of Newcastle schoolchildren in 1980. Less than one in eight of those children who turned out to have asthma had actually been so diagnosed. Then a London general practitioner, himself interested in asthma, was alarmed to find it often took his practice more than ten consultations before the penny dropped that they were seeing an asthmatic child. Subsequent surveys from Nottingham and elsewhere all point to the same conclusion. When survey teams specifically look for asthmatic children, they find at least one in ten have the condition. Yet only half of these have been diagnosed as asthmatic and receive correct treatment. Such figures translated into the reality of a school of 500 pupils, mean that for each of the 25 or so diagnosed asthmatics, there will be another 25 undiagnosed, untreated, and under performing on that account.

Asthmatic children for the most part minimize the severity of their illness, and do not like to be seen as different from their classmates. They are none the less upset by unsympathetic attitudes from other children or from their teachers, for example, over the use of inhalers. Despite the degree of under diagnosis, of all children requiring to take any sort of medication in school, two thirds of them are asthmatic. Clear understanding and guidelines about the use of asthma treatment in school are thus vital. Time off school as a result of asthma can be a real problem. Half of those diagnosed as asthmatic, and almost as many of those with undiagnosed asthma, will need to stay away from school for at least a day or two per year, and in the worst cases this will be a month or more. School absence in the asthmatic child (as for others) is influenced by home circumstances such as poor social conditions, large family, and low income, but for the most part reflects the severity of their asthma. It seems self-evident that closer attention to diagnosis and treatment by the child's GP and better understanding of their condition by teachers would lessen school absence and improve participation in games.

## The outlook for asthmatic children

There is a strongly held view that children 'grow out' of asthma. Reasons for supposing this might happen are not difficult to find. With growing up, the air passages of the lungs widen so that any degree of narrowing is less noticeable: allergies often seem better tolerated: and immunity develops to infection. But what is the truth of the matter? There have now been several quite long term follow-up studies of asthmatic children to see what happens to them in later life.

One of the earliest was by a London general practitioner, Dr Henry Blair. He reviewed over 200 asthmatics some 20 years after he had first met them in childhood. For convenience we can divide them into roughly equal quarters. A quarter had no asthma at the 20 year follow-up date: another quarter had very mild symptoms: and another quarter had persisting asthma requiring regular treatment. What about the remaining quarter? They had also become, at some stage, completely free of their asthma, and remained so for at least three years. However, after that their asthma had returned, not necessarily severely but sufficiently to require some treatment. Those tolerant Melbourne children mentioned earlier have also been re-examined at 28 years. It was reassuring to note that three quarters of those who were wheezy at age seven years had stopped being so by age 14 years, strongly supporting the 'growing out' story. But keeping an eye on these lucky ones over the next 14 years disappointingly showed that in about a half the asthma had come back again. Furthermore some of those who had only been mildly affected in childhood had deteriorated, so that overall there were still almost a quarter of these children with persisting symptoms, very similar to the proportion found by Dr Blair.

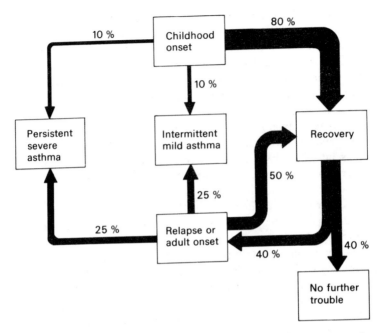

The outcome of asthma: very approximate figures based on several series from different countries.

This general trend has now been confirmed in surveys from New Zealand, Scandinavia, and the UK. So asthma does tend to go away, but it doesn't necessarily stay away. Recurrence later in life seems to remain a threat even for those with mild childhood asthma.

Enquiry into which children are more likely to have persistent symptoms reveals a cluster of so-called risk factors. Some we might guess from what we have learned already—early age of onset, higher frequency of attacks, presence of allergy and maternal smoking. But others are less obvious, such as being female, being born to a young mother, low birth weight, and high living standards.

## Asthma and hay fever

If children with asthma are monitored throughout childhood, the number giving positive tests for allergy increases, even though the extent to which they are bothered by asthma lessens. Hay fever symptoms also become more common early in the second decade of life. Hay fever beginning for the first time in an atopic child who has not previously had asthma is likely to do so in the early teenage years. Pollen asthma may accompany the hay fever as noted earlier. When it does, the asthma is often purely summer seasonal. Even so, it does not behave in an exclusively 'allergic' way. While the hay fever may come on immediately after exposure to pollen, the asthma rarely does. More often it appears in the familiar form of nocturnal wheezing attacks. As the season advances, the wheezing persists into the day, but exacerbations in a pollen-laden atmosphere are not prominent. Exercise, cold air, and irritant dusts may now set off wheezing, whereas in the winter these can be tolerated without ill effect. The pollen is clearly an essential factor in the development of the asthma, but it creates a state in which many triggers, not just allergy, will set up wheezing.

Hay fever and pollen asthma tend to be less and less bothersome by the late teenage years. Many other childhood asthmatics have 'grown out' of their asthma by this age. So, early adult life tends to be a period of life when asthma is less common. Those bothered by asthma at this stage include children whose symptoms have persisted through the teenage years and the few whose asthma begins for the first time at this age.

## Adult asthma

Asthma presents a more varied and less stereotyped picture in the adult, than that just described in children. Certainly there are many adults with a typical pattern of recurrent attacks of asthma, often triggered by allergy or infection, and with symptom-free intervals maintained by regular therapy. But in the adult there is a greater tendency for symptoms to become persistent and more difficult to control. Sometimes this takes the form of very variable wheezing, the lung function swinging wildly for weeks on end: for others there is a slowly progressive shortness of breath with variations in function becoming smaller and smaller, and response to treatment less striking. This latter trend is enhanced by the vice of cigarette smoking, still an unaccountably common habit among asthmatics.

Adults with asthma, whether it is intermittent or persistent, are unlikely to have or have had symptoms all their lives. In some their asthma has persisted from childhood through adolescence and into adult life: in others there has been a period of more or less complete absence of any symptoms for several years, even a decade or two until a relapse occurs. For some there is a mere hint of previous trouble—some 'wheezy bronchitis' or a little eczema or summer hay fever reflecting their tendency to allergies. For yet others, and these can represent up to 50% of all those who ever get asthma, symptoms begin for the first time in adult life. There is no dominant age in adult life for new asthma to start, and indeed it can appear—or certainly only be first recognized as important—in old age.

## Causes of asthma in adults

The circumstances which initiate or subsequently trigger asthma in adults are extremely varied. Careful attention to detail can reveal unexpected causes: equally in others no amount of probing can elucidate why attacks occur so that their asthma appears truly intrinsic.

The re-appearance or first occurrence of asthma in adult life should prompt, first, a search for a change in circumstances that has led to an encounter with *a new allergen*. This is most likely to be something that is breathed in—so a change of environment may be responsible: a new house, a new pet, a change of job. Environmental changes, relating to occupation, are discussed later (Chapter 8).

In the adult it is important to enquire about the *introduction of treatment* given for conditions other than asthma that might be responsible for initiating the appearance or recurrence of symptoms. Most important in this context are the *betablockers*. These drugs are used widely for high blood pressure, irregular heart beats, and some other conditions. Their effect, however, directly opposes certain treatments needed for asthma, so they can be dangerous for asthmatics even when only used as eye drops.

*Aspirin-induced asthma* is clearly recognizable but not common. It usually develops in young adults. Within a few minutes of taking aspirin, there is sneezing and running of the nose, followed quickly by tightness in the chest and wheezing. Repeated attacks lead to polyps forming in the nose and a rather persistent asthma. The probable reasons for all this were described earlier (Chapter 3). Asthmatics should be wary not only of aspirin but also of related tablets known as NSAIDs (non-steroidal anti-inflammatory drugs)—some of which, like Nurofen (ibuprofen) can be bought over the counter.

*Chest infections* are associated both with a first attack of asthma in the adult or its re-appearance after years of absence and with recurring attacks. This seems particularly so in those asthmatics who do not give positive skin prick tests for atopic allergy and thus are classified as 'intrinsic'. The story is often one of persistent coughing and wheezing initiated by an influenza-like illness. Several courses of antibiotics may be given with disappointing results. The illness does not respond until it is appreciated that there is a wheezy component and appropriate treatment prescribed. The same sequence follows another infection months later. The interval between infective wheezy episodes may shorten but this is not predictable. There may be persisting shortness of breath between attacks, with weather conditions appearing to be responsible for episodic chest tightness. Progression to a state of chronic disability occurs more frequently in these individuals than in childhood.

Besides infection, many adults rank *stress* as important in initiating or reactivating their asthma. Earning a living becomes more physically arduous. Family life brings its worries. The realities of life demand that ideals be compromised for practicalities. Some notice that it is not the stress itself but the relief from tension that comes after a particularly stressful time has passed, that initiates the asthma. A woman may develop wheezing after nursing her husband through a terminal illness. A man finds his job increasingly demanding yet is resentful when he is passed over for promotion: he too may become asthmatic. Individual case records can be very convincing. How specific these psychological stresses are in initiating asthma in the adult is debatable, and how they interact with other internal or external factors to trigger asthma is unknown. Periods of anxiety are not rare and it is tempting to attribute physical illness to stress.

A particular expression of stress can cause considerable confusion for doctors treating asthma in the sense that it sounds like asthma but in reality is not. Whistling wheezy sounds called stridor are made in the voice box (larynx) rather than coming from the small air passages in the lung (which remain clear). There is nothing structurally wrong with the larynx—and so the condition is called functional laryngeal stridor. It is distressing but not dangerous. It does not upset the efficiency with which oxygen gets through the lungs into the body. Unfortunately, large doses of asthma treatments are often mistakenly prescribed, and this can be detrimental. The condition is best treated by speech therapy and removing the cause of the stress.

There are a few *unusual forms of asthma* in adults that need mentioning. The first is exclusive to women. It is asthma that seems to coincide in time with their menstrual cycle being worse during the flow and just pre-menstrually. It is quite a common observation but the worsening is usually slight. In the occasional severe case, the female sex hormone, progesterone, has proved helpful treatment.

Many women with asthma are concerned how they will manage when pregnant. It is, in fact, quite unpredictable, save for noting that an attack of asthma in labour is exceptionally uncommon. In a few, their asthma may worsen during childbearing, in some it improves but for most pregnancy has no obvious effect on their asthma. Late in pregnancy the encumbrance of the large baby leads to some shortness of breath but this is not asthma.

Next there is asthma associated with a form of indigestion known as gastro-oesophageal reflux. In this, acid from the stomach regurgitates up into the swallowing tube (the oesophagus or gullet) which lies behind the breast bone. Not only does this cause a sharp pain but, in a way not really understood, it can make asthma worse. Treatment for the acid reflux can, in these instances, relieve the asthma. The situation is complicated by the fact that some tablets used to treat asthma (e.g. aminophylline) can make acid reflux worse.

It is in the adult age group that the particular form of allergic asthma described earlier (Chapter 4) as due to the fungus Aspergillus, is most likely to occur. The mould spores of Aspergillus are prone to cause not only attacks of wheezing but, by damaging the central air passages, much more persistent symptoms.

## Chronic asthma

Persistent narrowing of the air passages between attacks of asthma will cause some degree of shortness of breath on exertion, often without obvious wheezing. It may be first noticed as a failure to recover fully after a cold that has gone onto the chest, or after encountering a heavy exposure to an allergen. Spells of such persistent asthma may give way to periods of greater freedom during which the asthma is again truly intermittent. It is the aim of treatment to achieve just this. More severe degrees of persistent narrowing lead to a state in which shortness of breath and wheeze become more permanent features of the daily life of the asthmatic. A state of truly disabling shortness of breath curtailing activity and necessitating a complete change of lifestyle is well recognized but not common in asthma. Even in this state the potential for change, which is such a feature of asthma, remains, both as sudden, temporary tightening of the chest and in spells of much improved symptoms.

Deciphering why asthma becomes chronic has not proved easy and the answers we have are far from complete. In Chapter 4 we noted that some allergens in some individuals give late allergic reactions. Such reactions are associated with more persistent symptoms, more damage to the airways, and a greater tendency to chronic symptoms. Whilst the Aspergillus fungus is one clearly defined agent which is associated with damaging asthma, it is by no means the only one nor indeed the commonest. Other allergens can produce persistent asthma, but why they do not always do so, or why it is only a problem for some asthmatics is not known.

There is also a tendency towards persistent asthma in those asthmatics who smoke. Wheezing in the adult all too often presents a difficult diagnostic dilemma: is it asthma or is it wheeziness in someone with chronic bronchitis due to smoking? Some chronic bronchitics certainly develop narrowed airways. This narrowing is more permanent and progressive than that seen in ordinary asthma. But in some adults it is, at least initially, quite remarkably reversible. Infection is an important trigger for episodes of reversible wheeziness in the adult smoker. In these, the wheezy bronchitis has many parallels to the wheezy bronchitis seen in asthmatics. Some smokers develop wheezing because they are already asthmatic. Others have had some sort of childhood respiratory illness. In a fair proportion, the childhood illness must have been asthma or wheezy bronchitis. It is possible then to argue either that smoking is one of the factors likely to trigger asthma in those constitutionally predisposed to it, or that in smokers a previous history of asthma makes them more prone to the injurious effects of tobacco smoke.

## Late onset asthma

This is a loose term, not well defined, and may only mean that the asthma becomes recognized late in life, even though it has been present for some time. For the most part, asthma that starts late in life is not allergic and really it equates with intrinsic asthma as described earlier. It is not often appreciated that asthma can appear for the first time in the elderly. In those over 65 years, asthma is diagnosed in only about

5–6% but, as with children, there is probably serious under diagnosis. On the basis of having a low peak flow test that responds to asthma treatments, up to a third of the elderly fit the bill. Unless they have previously been known to have asthma, wheezing shortness of breath in those over 65 years of age is more likely to be attributed to the effects of smoking or to some other chest or heart condition. Yet surveys show that quite a number of elderly people do indeed have genuine asthma. When asthma does develop in the elderly, infection is very likely to be a factor in both initiating the illness and in triggering subsequent attacks. Persistent symptoms, with a need for continuous medication and a progressive course, are unfortunately likely to be the outlook.

## Inheritance

Those with asthma often ask whether they are likely to pass the disorder on to their children. It is a question to which we are beginning to find the answer. There is no doubt that asthma 'runs in families'. In 1650, Sennertus described it in three successive generations of his wife's family. Working out how asthma is inherited or what chance there is that a given individual will develop asthma, is one of the most exciting areas in current asthma research.

Our modern understanding of genetics, the science of inheritance, began with Gregor Mendel, born into a poor Austrian peasant family in 1822. He became a priest, and in 1858, abbot of the monastery at Brno in the present day Czech Republic. There, he carried out his painstaking crossbreeding experiments. They revealed that some characteristics were dominant, appearing in the offspring whether they received the genetic signal from both or from just one parent. Other characteristics were recessive and appeared only when inherited from both parents. In animals such simple rules explained the inheritance of eye and fur colour. For other characteristics, such as height or blood pressure, several different genetic signals seem to be necessary, since the inheritance cannot be explained by applying simple Mendelian rules.

How do the rules apply to asthma? The first step was to realize that it is necessary to look beyond asthma as such, to allergy in general. Indeed we have to consider all of that group of allergic disorders that we earlier described as atopic—infantile eczema, hay fever, and urticaria (hives) as well as asthma. Early surveys suggested that in about half of any group of patients with these allergies, there was a family history of asthma. In other words it was 'the tendency to develop allergy' that seemed to be inherited rather than any particular allergic condition.

With the development of tests for allergy, like skin tests and measuring the allergic antibody in the blood, it has now become possible to build up a composite picture of the allergic status of an individual. Using this approach Julian Hopkin and his team in Oxford have begun to define how the tendency to develop allergy is inherited. These researchers looked first at simple family groups consisting of one child and two parents. Selecting twenty children with asthma and twenty of similar age who had some entirely unrelated condition, such as appendicitis, they have found a remarkable difference between the parents. In nineteen out of the twenty pairs of parents of the asthmatic children, at least one parent was found to be allergic compared with only six of the twenty pairs of parents of the other children. This finding points to dominant inheritance according to Mendel's rules. Looking at very large families confirmed this view. Some families contained over one hundred people: all of them were traced and studied. The characteristics that defined the tendency to develop allergy could be seen passing down from one generation to the next. It is important to realize that not all these allergic people had a recognizable condition. Though some were asthmatic and others may have had hay fever, some had no obvious allergic disorder at all, just the tendency revealed in their blood and skin tests to be capable of developing allergy.

The instructions our bodies follow to create blue eyes or blonde hair or the tendency to develop allergy are contained in tiny fragments called genes. We possess about 100 000 genes. They are strung together in minute filaments called chromosomes, which themselves are joined together, like an X, in 21 pairs. The chromosomes themselves are packaged together inside the centre or nucleus of every cell in our bodies. When research suggests a particular disorder is inherited, the next step is for the scientist to search amongst all the genes to see if they can identify the particular one that carries the message that leads to the development of that particular disorder. It really is very much like looking for a needle in a hay stack.

How far have we reached in finding the allergy gene? Quite a long way. First, it has been discovered that a most important gene responsible for the tendency to develop allergy lies on chromosome number 11: secondly, it is only active when it is inherited from the mother: and thirdly, it only accounts for about one

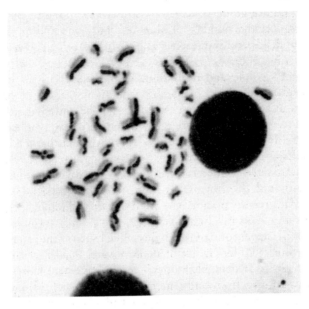

Human chromosomes.

half of examples of allergic inheritance, so other genes must exist elsewhere.

It is exciting to be able to say that the first report of an identified genetic abnormality in a group of allergic individuals has now been published. The gene determines our response to the allergic antibody, IgE (see Chapter 4) and a small, but potentially crucial, change in the gene has been discovered. The change is very likely to be responsible for their tendency to be allergic. What does this mean? Once a gene is identified in this way it can be studied to find out just what it does in the body. Revealing how differently the abnormal gene behaves will enable us to devise treatments that will restore its function to normal, so hopefully restoring those with it to a state in which they are no longer prone to allergies. Already other genes are being identified which are abnormal in other asthmatics leading to the prospect of more specific treatments tailored to the needs of different individuals.

Whilst the manner in which allergy is inherited is becoming clearer, the inheritance of asthma is rather more complex. For example, most children who are going to develop asthma have done so by the age of 5 years. Yet the number of skin test positive children increases throughout childhood and reaches its peak in the teens. This divergence between asthma and atopic allergies can be picked up in detailed family studies. Both atopic and non-atopic asthmatics show an increased family incidence of asthma. It is somewhat more marked in the atopic asthmatics. It seems that being atopic allows the underlying tendency to asthma to express itself more easily. Atopy is certainly inherited but not necessarily together with asthma. There is a hint that the inherited asthmatic trait is the irritable nature of the airways. Some relatives of asthmatics respond to exercise with airways narrowing in an asthmatic way even though they themselves have never wheezed.

Whatever precise explanations for the inheritance of asthma and allergy emerge from this line of research, it is clear that we are going to have to understand not only the inheritance but also the interaction of that individual with his environment. Exposures to allergens, infection, and other environmental hazards are clearly important in determining the extent to which the inherited tendency to asthma and allergy is expressed. It is possible to gain some further insight into the relationships between inheritance and environment in asthma by taking a yet broader view of asthma. This will be done in the next two chapters.

# 8 *Asthma and the environment*

Environmental issues have never been of greater public concern. A threat is perceived to the very future of the planet. Such a grand perspective is beyond the scope of a modest text on asthma, but the impact of the environment on the lives of asthmatics most certainly is not.

So far, we have seen, in earlier chapters, how specific external triggers cause asthma, and how internal and inherent factors modify how asthma affects people of different ages. This chapter looks at the environment we live in, to see how it impacts on asthmatics. We shall need to consider homes, places of work, climate, and pollution. Each has a different story to tell, but common themes tie them together.

## The domestic environment

The name of the house dust mite signals its importance in our homes. How this microscopic creature behaves was considered earlier (Chapter 4). We are responsible for the dust mite being such an important domestic allergen. We warm our homes to a temperature it enjoys; we close the windows, so creating a dampness it can thrive in; we fill our homes with soft bedding and thick carpets, which provide it a fertile breeding ground. No wonder one in five of us shows evidence of allergy to the mite. We are responsible too for bringing animals, especially cats and dogs into our homes. We create the allergic environment which will lead the genetically susceptible individual to develop asthma.

Besides these well-recognized allergens, most other features of the domestic scene are relatively unimportant. Moulds in damp houses can produce allergy, though less frequently than the Aspergillus found in compost heaps in the garden. There is also a curious allergic reaction to formaldehyde used in the manufacture of chipboard. Built into the walls, especially it seems, of mobile homes, this gives off fumes which in rare instances have caused asthma.

Other fumes do not act allergically. Gas cookers give off a gas known as nitrogen dioxide (this crops up again later when we consider car exhaust pollution). There is a clear association between the actual levels of nitrogen dioxide in the home and both breathing complaints and breathing tests. Children who live in homes where gas cookers are used are up to twice as likely to develop asthma. Comments have been made earlier (Chapter 7) about the increased risk to children who live in homes where there are smokers—especially a smoking mother. And the two risks often occur together. Though not in themselves causes of asthma, the fumes given off by gas cookers and the spare smoke from cigarettes seem to interact with allergens and genetic susceptibility in encouraging the development of asthma.

Outside the home, a great deal of attention has been focused on what happens at work as a cause of asthma.

## Occupational asthma

Occupational medicine was created almost overnight by the publication in 1700 of the book *De Morbus Artificum Diatribe*. It records the painstaking observations of one man, Bernadino Ramazzini of Modena. It is a classic. He enquired into the working conditions of potters, tinsmiths, tanners, cheesemakers, stonecutters, grooms, farmers, and countless others, and concluded: 'Medicine, like jurisprudence, should make a contribution to the wellbeing of workers . . . To the questions recommended by Hippocrates add one more—What is your occupation?'

Only some of the complaints described by Ramazzini were asthmatic. In the twentieth century the ever-increasing diversity of industrial processes using chemicals, creating vapours, and raising dusts has vastly multiplied the opportunities for the lungs to react to inhaled agents by producing asthma. The detective work involved in tracking down the responsible agents is always fascinating. And the potential for cure exists by the use of simple techniques of industrial hygiene.

What clues should alert to the possibility of occupational asthma? Asthma coming on for the first time in a working adult. Asthma that is present during the week but clears up at weekends or on holiday. Sometimes there will be a very obvious relation to some particular process, such as soldering, colour printing, or preparing chemicals. Sometimes the symptoms will initially be running of the nose, or watering of the eyes, and only later will there be coughing and wheezing.

The relationship between work and asthma can—and should—be confirmed by measurements of peak flow. A series of tests, if possible every two hours during the day, will detect asthma developing during the working day, and fail to show it at the weekend or on holiday. A typical chart is shown, simplified to show average morning and evening readings only.

The name given to a substance encountered at work which gives rise to asthma is a sensitizer. The circumstances of exposure to the sensitizing agent are important. Length of time in the industry is a very crude index. Even with a single agent this timing is exceedingly variable. Some workers develop wheezing within a few months—others not for years. The degree of exposure—concentration of dust or vapour—whether it is intermittent or continuous—whether there is sufficient ventilation—where the workers stand or sit in the factory—all these and many other external factors influence whether or not asthma will develop.

Occupational asthmas can arise from environmental pollution. One factory recognizing that its processes were generating chemicals likely to cause asthma, fitted a ventilation system. The dust from this poured through the windows of the factory next door and the workers there developed asthma.

There is now a huge list of industries in which some process or other has been implicated in the causation of occupational asthma. Lists of some of the commoner ones are given. The interaction between

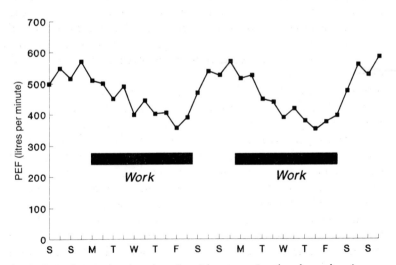

Peak flow changes in an asthmatic with occupational asthma showing progressive worsening during the working week and recovery at the weekend.

the host—(the asthmatic worker)—and the sensitizing agent (dust, chemical, and so on) is often revealing and worth following through.

---

**Organic agents**

| *Occupation* | *Agents implicated* |
| --- | --- |
| Animal handlers | Hair, dander, mites, insects |
| Bakers | Flour dust, moulds, weevils |
| Coffee industry | Green coffee dust |
| Cotton workers | Cotton, flax, hemp |
| Detergent industry | Proteolytic enzymes |
| Domestics etc. | House dust |
| Electricians | Soldering fluxes |
| Oil extractors | Castor bean, linseed, and cotton seed |
| Pharmaceutical industry | Penicillin and other antibiotics, piperazine sulphonamides |
| Poultry workers | Feathers |
| Printers | Gum arabic, tragacanth |
| Wood workers | Dust from western red cedar, Iroko etc. |

---

## Occupational allergy to organic material

First and simplest, some subjects may find themselves encountering unduly frequently simple environmental allergens to which any atopic asthmatic might react. Domestics and factory cleaners will raise dusts containing the ubiquitous 'house' dust mite. Jockeys, shepherds, and vets will handle horses, sheep, cats, and other animals and may show asthmatic reactions to hair or skin dander. Laboratory workers handle other animals and, whilst these are not common allergens, the principle is the same. Locusts are highly sensitizing: so is the urine of rats and mice. All these are allergens of organic origin, in other words they come from living things such as animals or plants.

The work of *bakers* illustrates how complex allergic asthma can be in the occupational setting, even when none other than naturally occurring allergens have to be considered. To many with established asthma the fine dust of flour is a simple irritant capable of setting up reflex bronchospasm. The flour can act as an allergen too. Atopic sensitivity to flour, demonstrable by positive skin prick tests is frequent. Flour and grain left standing, invite unwanted visitors. Moulds such as

*Aspergillus* and *Penicillium*, the grain weevil *Sitophilus granularis*, and storage mites can all create allergic asthma.

Allergic occupational asthmas like these occur more frequently in atopic people—indeed the sufferers may already have, or have had, asthma. The issue of smoking cigarettes comes into the picture again. Sensitivity to the colophony resin used in soldering in the electronics industry is several times more likely to produce asthmatic symptoms in a smoker as it is in a non-smoker. Similar trends occur with other causes of occupational asthma.

---

### Inorganic agents

| | |
|---|---|
| Chemical workers | Formalin, isocyanates; phthalic anhydride and epoxy resins |
| Meat packers | Fumes from polyvinyl film cut with hot wire |
| Metal workers | Nickel, vanadium, chromium |
| Paint workers | Toluene di-isocyanates |
| Photographic industry | Complex salts of platinum |
| Rubber industry | Ethylene diamine and paraphenylene diamine |

---

## Occupational asthma due to inorganic material

Other sensitizing agents are inorganic, in other words they don't come from living things of any sort. A useful list is included in the table. Under appropriate circumstances occupational asthma can be caused by these substances irrespective of whether the individual is atopic or not. Two of these are worth considering, in a little detail, the first because of its historic interest, and the second because it is the commonest form of occupational asthma experienced in this country.

The precious silvery-white metal *platinum*, when used in industry in the form of complex chloride salts, produces asthma in 100% of workers exposed to it for five years or more. Those involved in extracting the metal and preparing its salts are most at risk but there is danger, too, to those working in electroplating workshops, in photographic studios using plate toning, and in jewellers.

An allergic basis for platinum asthma is strongly suggested by the pattern of challenge tests—both immediate, late, and double reactions are recorded. Skin prick tests, too, are positive and antibodies have been found in the blood, so supporting the proposal that this is truly an allergic asthma.

The situation with isocyanates is less clear cut. These chemicals have the dubious distinction of being the commonest cause of occupational asthma, being responsible for one fifth of the compensated cases. Initially introduced in the manufacture of polyurethane foams, they are now widely used for making adhesives, synthetic rubbers, and especially, spray paints for cars. Toluene di-isocyanate (TDI) is the compound most often used. It is highly volatile and a potent trigger for respiratory symptoms.

The fumes of TDI are undoubtedly directly irritant to the nose, throat, and chest. Regular exposure to concentrations released during normal manufacturing processes can set up an irritating cough and asthmatic wheezing. On leaving the industry, sufferers mostly recover very quickly. However, in a few, subsequent exposure to very small concentrations of TDI has led, once more, to asthmatic wheezing. This observation suggests allergy: but proof has been difficult to come by. Whilst challenge tests are usually positive, skin prick tests and blood allergy tests give inconsistent results. Atopy does not predispose to the development of isocyanate asthma, but previous asthma does.

With TDI it is worth remembering that exposure can occur outside the actual manufacturing industry. Polyurethane foam 'do-it-yourself' kits have been marketed. Much more subtle is the exposure of previously sensitized subjects to small concentrations of TDI, when polyurethane foam is cut or crushed in the hand.

## Lessons to be learned from occupational asthma

While occupational asthmas hold much of interest for those involved with the management of this disorder, perhaps three points stand out beyond any others. The first concerns the nature of atopic allergy. Atopic sensitivity to commonly encountered environmental allergens is found in about one in three of the general population. But it emerges from the study of occupational asthmas that heavy exposure to certain allergens—of which locusts and the complex salts of platinum seem to be good examples—can produce atopic sensitivity both in the skin and in the airways in much higher proportion of the exposed population.

Secondly, the occupational asthmas confirm the impression given by some other allergic asthmas that a combination of immediate and late asthmatic reactions is quite common. This goes a long way towards reconciling the differences between naturally occurring asthma—in which attacks last many hours or even days—and challenge tests, which if confined to a consideration of immediate reactions are all over in a couple of hours.

Thirdly, the potential for cure exists more realistically in relation to the occupational asthmas than it does in respect to any other form of asthma. Even for this reason alone they require the most careful analysis and investigation.

## Compensation for occupational asthma

Asthma developing as a result of occupational exposure was first recognized as a compensatable hazard in the 1960s in France and Germany. In Britain compensation under the Industrial Injuries Act became possible in 1981 for certain specific exposures. The list was reviewed at intervals, but became so long that in 1991 the rules were changed. Benefit is now payable whatever the cause provided the Benefits Officer is satisfied that occupational asthma has been firmly diagnosed. A worsening of pre-existing asthma by working conditions is not normally compensatable, but any asthmatics who feel that their symptoms have only come on in relation to specific working conditions should first consult their general practitioner. Appropriate tests can then be advised before submitting a claim to the local office of the Department of Health and Social Security.

## The weather and pollution

Many patients would argue the importance of the weather in triggering asthmatic attacks. Damp and cold feature prominently. Coastland dwellers gain relief by moving inland where it is warmer and drier. A drop in air temperature will upset some asthmatics: others will say they like cold, crisp days. Hot and humid weather is often disliked; yet warm, moist air can prevent exercise-induced asthma. At first sight nothing seems to hang together, so we need to look more carefully at what observations are available.

In casualty departments worldwide, careful records show that emergency attendances by asthmatics at night vary with temperature and humidity. A sharp drop in atmospheric temperature, often with the formation of mist or fog, seems to set off a spate of asthma attacks. But there is also a more general increase in asthma associated with the damp autumnal and winter months. What is going on? A simple explanation in terms of cold air tightening the chest doesn't seem enough. It could be that the cold weather drives the asthmatic indoors where he or she is more continuously exposed to house dust allergens. Perhaps on the other hand it is the occurrence of viral chest infections, encouraged by the weather conditions, that is important.

Other short-lived epidemics of asthma occur in association with sudden heavy rainfall. The water breaks up pollen grains and mould spores, releasing them into the atmosphere. These will trigger off asthma in sensitive individuals. But it is the combination of climatic change with atmospheric pollutants that has excited most interest.

Starting with an account of asthma in New Orleans, there have now been reported some remarkable outbreaks of asthma in large cities, clustered in the summer months. These are attacks of genuine asthma, mostly in previously known asthmatics. Meteorological analysis associates the outbreaks with hot days, low wind speed, low relative humidity, and a drop in temperature at night. Such circumstances trap air in an almost motionless layer over the city. Allergens and pollutants build up in the stagnant air and the city's asthmatics succumb. Pollution has become a hotly debated issue for asthmatics. We need to examine it cooly.

The atmosphere is not just a vehicle for climatic change. Air pollution, of local importance in occupational asthma, is of general importance and concern when it contaminates the environment of whole cities. Sulphur dioxide is one well recognized culprit, and a powerful irritant to the bronchial tree. The airways tighten within ten seconds of inhaling it. Respiratory disease in a community can be correlated with the amount of sulphur dioxide in the atmosphere: asthmatics have more attacks: bronchitics wheeze more readily.

Pollutants come chiefly from the burning of fossil fuels, coal, diesel, and petrol. Experience in Britain following the introduction of the Clean Air Act showed that the atmosphere of our cities could be made cleaner and clearer. The particles of soot and dense sulphurous fumes that contributed to the infamous smogs of the 1950s largely disappeared, though similar improvements are awaited in the highly polluted industrial zones of other parts of the world. Yet whilst bronchitis and chest infections have decreased as a result, asthma has not. Although the visible pollution has disappeared, gaseous pollution has not. In addition there has been a vast increase in road traffic, and traffic produces exhaust fumes. Amongst other things, these fumes contain oxides of nitrogen which in the right climatic conditions lead to the formation of ozone.

So the pollutants we need to consider are:

- Smoke; no longer do we see large black pieces of soot but there are still small particles chiefly coming from diesel engines. They are known as $PM_{10}$s (particulate matter of 10 microns size, or less).

- Sulphur dioxide ($SO_2$): there is still some of this coming from power stations.

- Nitrogen dioxide ($NO_2$): this is on the increase. Vehicle fuels produce nitric oxide which changes to $NO_2$ in the atmosphere.

- Ozone ($O_3$) this is formed by the action of sunlight on $NO_2$.*

These gases, especially $SO_2$ but also ozone and to a small degree $NO_2$, are directly irritant to the lungs. They cause cough, wheeze, and narrowed airways.

But what is the evidence that these pollutants have anything to do with asthma? There are two lines of investigation that lend support to there being a link between atmospheric pollution and asthma. First are comparisons made between records of attendances at hospital and simultaneous records of specific pollutants. In Canada, in France, in England and indeed elsewhere, admissions for asthma are higher when levels of atmospheric ozone, $SO_2$, $NO_2$, and $PM_{10}$ rise. The second line of evidence comes from challenge studies in individuals (like those described in Chapter 3 for histamine and methacholine). Asthmatics are more sensitive than others to sulphur dioxide and to combinations of $SO_2$ with ozone and nitrogen dioxide.

But there is another strand to the story. In Japan some surprise was expressed when allergy to cedar pollen (especially sneezing but also asthma) was found more commonly in town dwellers who lived along cedar lined highways, than in those living in the countryside where there were just as many cedar trees. The finger pointed again at the car fumes. This inspired a series of studies combining allergen challenge with pollutant exposure. If asthmatics breathe low levels of a pollutant gas before they are challenged with an allergen, then they get a bigger reaction than if the pollutant is omitted. This interaction has now been

* Ozone is an important part of the atmosphere. Indeed high up it is essential to shield us from the effects of ultraviolet light and we all know of concern over the Antarctic ozone hole. The ozone from car exhausts is of no help—it's down at ground level, and too much at that level is harmful.

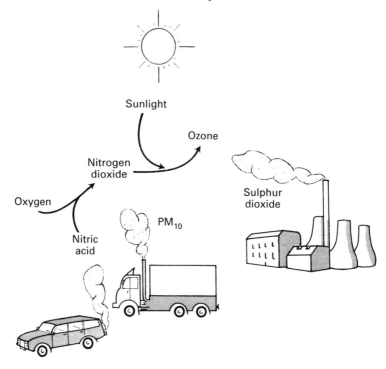

The origins of atmospheric pollution.

documented for ragweed pollen with ozone, and for house dust mite with $SO_2$ and with $SO_2$ and $NO_2$ combined.

Thus it all begins to fit together. Asthmatics have irritable airways. They are irritable because they are inflamed. They are inflamed because of the effects of allergy, the effects of infection, the effects of pollution. But rarely does one act alone. The effect of allergen is worse in the presence of pollutants, the effect of an occupational hazard is worse in the smoker. The effect of the viral infection is worse in the allergic individual and so on.

This chapter has broadened our view of asthma by looking at wider environmental issues than those which affect single individuals. It leads on to a world view of asthma and introduces the idea of studying large populations as a means of increasing our understanding of this fascinating disorder.

# 9 *Asthma worldwide*

Clues to the causation of illness can often be picked up by taking a global rather than a parochial view. Malaria is only contracted in certain parts of the world. These parts are generally hot and humid. It turns out that climate influences malaria by providing appropriate breeding conditions for the *Anopheles* mosquito. Through the bite of this insect, malaria is passed on from one person to another. The analysis of such environmental conditions has contributed immeasurably to the discovery of the causes of many of the major epidemic illnesses of the world.

This approach, which began as a study of epidemics of infectious diseases, which from time to time sweep across the globe, has long since extended its horizons to look at non-infectious diseases. Epidemiology is concerned with the pattern of diseases on a larger scale than that observable in single patients. The pattern of diseases in families, in groups, and in races, is examined to determine the frequency with which the disorder is seen, the age range of afflicted persons and the personal, climatic, and environmental factors that seem to be associated with the disease under study. Epidemiological research can be applied to asthma. From this research some fascinating facts emerge, but before lining these up for appraisal, some cautionary notes must be sounded.

First, for sensible and reliable answers to any questions about asthma, the condition must be defined accurately. Regrettably this has not always been so in epidemiological studies of asthma. To be fair, the difficulties are formidable. They centre around the dilemma of detail versus numbers. The stricter the criteria used to define asthma, the more elaborate needs to be the questioning and testing. This takes time and personnel, and means that limits are set on the number of subjects that can be assessed. On the other hand, epidemiological research is best served by studying large numbers of people. Indeed best of all served by questioning everyone in a given community. The definition of asthma under these circumstances may have to rely on nothing more than the questions 'Do you have asthma?' or 'Do you have wheezing?' The answer to the first of these questions will depend not only on what the person being questioned believes about asthma, but also on what their doctor considers is asthma, and how much he has communicated his opinion to his patient. Wheezing, although an important audible accompaniment of asthma, occurs as noted earlier in other conditions and so may be less reliable in guiding epidemiological research than is a question about asthma itself.

If the first danger concerns the definition of asthma, the second concerns timing. Asthma, by its nature, is an intermittent disorder. So the question 'do you have asthma?' must be qualified: 'Do you have asthma today?' or 'Have you had asthma at any time in your life?' The answers to these questions give two figures for the frequency of asthma. Both are termed a prevalence. The first will be a point prevalence referring to all cases of asthma identified as present on the day the study is carried out. The second is a cumulative prevalence and includes in addition, those who might have seasonal asthma or who were asthmatic as children. Intermediate between these two is a period prevalence in which all those having asthma within a specified period are recorded.

The third danger in looking for epidemiological clues is more subtle. It concerns what other information should be gathered beyond the answers to the questions giving a prevalence figure. These questions depend on the preconceptions of the investigator. So the emphasis placed and the details recorded of climate, of industrialization, of race, of social class and custom, of environmental allergens, and so forth, will vary from survey to survey. The extent to which this information is recorded will colour and determine the conclusions that can be drawn from the study.

With these reservations in mind, what questions can we expect these large scale epidemiological studies to ask? First, and simplest, we can find out how many people have asthma. If that sort of survey is repeated, we can find out if, with the passage of time, more people or fewer people are getting asthma. Studies carried out in different parts of the world can pinpoint differences in asthma prevalence in different places. Then, by observing population movement we can ask whether it is the environment that seems to be responsible for the asthma, or whether it is some feature of the individuals themselves. Thus we can begin to explore the causes of asthma, not at an individual level, but in whole populations. Epidemiology is also used to examine the issues surrounding death from asthma.

## Asthma prevalence in the UK

Surveys of UK schoolchildren conducted over the last 5–10 years, all point to the quite startling fact that just over one child in ten has asthma—indeed most figures are closer to 12%, more like one in eight. Furthermore, framing the question as, 'wheeze at any time in childhood', produces figures more like 20% or one in five. In some of these compilations, only half of those with asthma (the 10–12%) were actually properly diagnosed and receiving appropriate treatment, though this proportion is showing signs of improvement.

In the first edition of *Asthma: the facts* (published in 1979), the figure given for the prevalence of asthma in UK children was only 2–4%. Has the number of asthmatics really increased? Or is it just that we are better able to recognize the condition, or more inclined to call any wheeziness, asthma? Careful repeat studies point clearly to a true increase. In children in South Wales asthma prevalence doubled over 15 years. Similarly in Aberdeen between 1964 and 1989 diagnosed asthma increased 2½ times and wheeze doubled.

Interestingly there have been similar recorded increases in other allergic disorders such as eczema and hay fever. Hay fever has changed its status during the twentieth century from being a medical curiosity, to a commonplace disorder. Nearly four times as many Aberdeen children had hay fever in 1989 compared with 1964 and in South Wales whilst only 5% of children had eczema in 1973, 16% suffered from it in 1988. The UK national study of children's health has confirmed all these trends, asthma rising from 4% in 1964 to 10% in 1989, and hay fever from 3% to 12%.

What can be happening? To attempt to answer that question we need to look at asthma prevalence beyond these shores.

## Worldwide asthma prevalence

Asthma is certainly not equally common in all parts of the world. In the highlands of Papua New Guinea asthma is so rare that the local population have no word for it. On Tristan da Cunha almost half the islanders give a history of asthma. Between these extremes, lie the developed countries like the UK and USA.

Setting aside the question of the definition of asthma and the type of prevalence recorded, the influences that can give rise to variations on a scale such as this are various, but they can be grouped together under two broad headings: nature and nurture. Nature is the inherited genetic make-up, which in its broadest sense means racial origin, and which, for the individual, means the family characteristics handed on from parents to children. Nurture implies environmental influence whether this be the effects of cultural habits and lifestyle, or external factors such as climate or exposure to allergens.

The populations which appear at the two extremes of the prevalence list tend to be highly inbred. Of the 15 original settlers on the remote south Atlantic island of Tristan da Cunha, three had asthma. All three were women, two from St. Helena and one from England. The volcano on Tristan da Cunha erupted in 1961 and the islanders were temporarily resettled in Britain. Medical checks emphasized the very high prevalence of asthma. The point prevalence—the number of cases actually wheezing on the day they were examined—was as high as 29% for the adults and 12% for the children. The change in environment to this country brought the islanders no relief from their persistent asthma. The islanders did not appear to be highly allergic, and investigations revealed no provoking agent present on Tristan da Cunha that could not be found elsewhere. Indeed, the commonest allergen was the ubiquitous house dust mite. Infection did commonly trigger their asthma but their minimal contact with the rest of the world meant that epidemics of infection occurred sporadically, brought in by visitors from passing ships. Psychological stress was not a feature of island life. So there is no escape from the conclusion that the islanders had inherited a tendency to asthma from their forebears which had been intensified by inbreeding.

There are lessons to be learnt, too, from places where asthma is uncommon, for example, the highlands of Papua New Guinea. How important genetic factors are in determining this low prevalence is less easy to discover. The indigenous population of Papua New Guinea are primitive people whose racial and cultural characteristics have remained unchanged for centuries. They have been and, for the most part, still are highly inbred. There are other primitive peoples who have similarly low figures: American Indians and the Eskimos. In Northern Canada only three Eskimos were admitted to hospital for asthma over a period of 12 years. The estimated prevalence rate was 0.08%—one in 1200.

The natives of Papua New Guinea and the Eskimos are unlikely to have much genetic material in common. They certainly do not share similar climatic conditions. But some parallels can be drawn between the

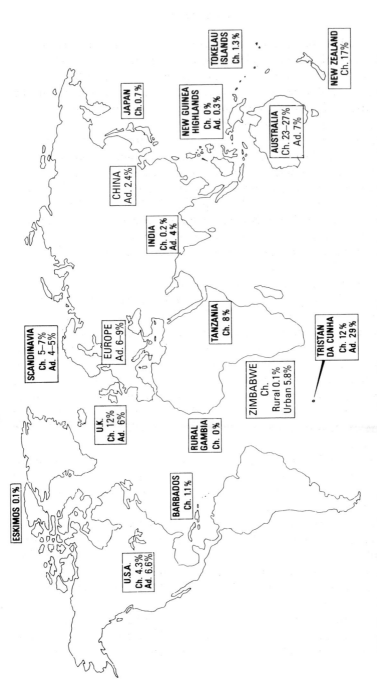

Worldwide prevalence of asthma: very approximate figures based on reported point and cumulative prevalences. Ch = children, Ad = adult.

lifestyles of these two communities. Perhaps the greatest amongst these might be their basically rural economy and lack of industrialization. It is of interest that in the last few years there has been a definite increase in asthma in Papua New Guinea, which appears to run parallel with the opening up of the country to Western influences. In particular allergic sensitivity to the house dust mite has appeared, whereas previously it was unknown. The bringing in of blankets harbouring the mite seems one likely source together with changes in housing which have encouraged it to breed.

An influence from urbanization seems to play a part in the prevalence of asthma in the west African state of the Gambia. Asthma is virtually unknown amongst villagers from rural communities. Just one case was on the files in a community of 1200. Yet in a town only 50 miles away, the hospital treated eight cases of asthma each day. Likewise, in urban populations from Kenya, Ghana, Zambia, and Nigeria asthma would appear to be a common problem. A recent detailed survey from Zimbabwe made this trend very obvious. In rural Wedza asthma prevalence was as low as 0.1%. In Harare, poor children recorded 3.1% asthma, whilst in the high socio-economic groups living in northern parts of the town, prevalence was up to 5.8% with no difference between white and black children. A breakdown of prevalence between urban and rural communities in western countries generally does not suggest anything like the striking differences recorded in less developed parts of the world. However, a survey of children from the Bronx area of New York recorded a one year prevalence of asthma of 8.6%, twice the general rate for US children. Cumulative prevalence was higher in children of Hispanic origin and those from low-income families.

Even within the developed world the prevalence of asthma is far from uniform. Two comparisons have been made between children in New Zealand and the UK. In almost all measures New Zealand children fared worse—more diagnosed asthma, more exercise-induced asthma, more wheezing by a factor of 1½ to 2 times. One of the studies, but not the other, recorded hospital admissions to be slightly fewer in New Zealand. Overall prevalences in Australia are also higher than the UK: but in the USA they are lower. Lifestyle differences must be minimal between these countries. Climate is clearly different but not in a consistent way. Patterns of health care are different and could be important.

## Population migration

The movement of people from a place with a low prevalence of asthma into urban communities offers interesting but not totally concordant information. Australasia provides another example. When the Tokelau Islands in the southern Pacific were hit by a hurricane, facilities were made available for the setting up of a Tokelau community in Wellington, New Zealand. The migrants began to complain increasingly of asthma. A careful survey showed that the Tokelau children living in New Zealand had twice as much asthma as those who had remained in their native islands, and very much more eczema.

Birmingham schoolchildren of all races were carefully surveyed for asthma by Dr Morrison-Smith. Negro children born in the West Indies have a lower prevalence of asthma than Caucasian children born in the United Kingdom. But West Indian children born in the UK have a similar prevalence to UK Caucasian children. Is the influence urbanization or something else connected with western civilization? Asian children born in India also have a lower prevalence of asthma than UK Caucasian children. But here the comparison fails. Asian children born in the UK do not show an increase in asthma as the West Indian children do or as the Tokelau Islanders did. Could this be because Asian families are less closely integrated into the local urban communities?

## Living in towns

A pattern begins to emerge. There seems to be some factor in urbanization, that allows asthma to become more common. This prompts a search for factors in the urban environment that might be responsible.

Returning first to Africa, a chance observation provoked a search for some link between parasitic diseases and asthma. British naval officers stationed in the Gambia reported less hay fever at times when they developed parasitic infections. In rural Africans, worm infestation is common: in the towns it is less so. The implication was drawn that the urban population in ridding themselves of intestinal parasites, at the same time became more liable to asthma.

Another possible explanation is related to cultural habits. Movement of peoples from a rural to an urban way of life is often associated with a decrease in the extent to which children are breast fed. In the first 6 months of life the child's chief nourishment is from milk. If the mother's milk is replaced by cows' milk, the exposure of the infant to foreign and potentially allergenic protein material will be increased. It does appear that avoidance of cows' milk by atopic children greatly reduces their chances of developing eczema. In view of the close association between eczema and asthma in infants, it was hoped that breastfeeding would reduce the chances of the children of allergic parents developing asthma. Regrettably this does not seem to be so.

An alternative idea, that would fit some of these observations, is that it is not the lack of mother's milk or even the introduction of cows' milk, but the exposure to other dietary agents, that has caused the increase in asthma. Certainly processed and packaged foods often contain a host of additives and preservatives that could potentially cause asthma and lack, in particular, Vitamin C that can protect against allergic inflammation.

Social differences apart from the question of breastfeeding, have at times figured in the asthma story. It was at one time suggested that children from the upper social classes were more prone to asthma, but careful study showed this not to be the case. Social class is, however, reflected in housing conditions and this may be a more relevant association.

## The rising prevalence of asthma

We are now in a position to return to the surprising, indeed alarming observations that point to a rising prevalence of asthma. Figures for the United Kingdom were quoted earlier; but similar trends are evident in Australia, New Zealand, Scandinavia, and the United States. The rising prevalence reflects itself not only in the answers to questionnaires but also in consultation rates to family doctors, attendances at emergency departments, and admissions to hospital. Various explanations have been put forward. None is entirely satisfactory but all are thought provoking.

### Better recognition

Doctors have been trained to recognize asthma better and parents have become much more aware of the condition. Illnesses previously called wheezy bronchitis are now labelled asthma. Improved medicines encourage more frequent diagnosis. Yet whilst this can explain some change, it does not account for the rising prevalences in communities where the same teams, using the same methods have conducted identical studies many years apart.

## Greater exposure to allergens

This is an attractive idea and fits in with the migration studies. Our homes are designed in a way that encourages growth of the house dust mite. Our children probably spend more time indoors in their cosy centrally heated bedrooms playing computer games. More and more allergens and sensitizers are recognized in the work place. Good information on the amount of allergen exposure over the years is, however, lacking, so it has been difficult to prove this idea.

## Pollution

There is no doubt, as we saw in Chapter 8, that pollution in our cities, particularly when combined with allergen exposure, precipitates attacks in those already known to have asthma. But can this account for the rise in asthma? Almost certainly not. It may encourage symptoms to persist for longer. This would make prevalence figures somewhat higher. There is no evidence that it creates more asthmatics.

Two observations are especially damaging to the pollution idea. First, the rising prevalence is found equally in remote rural districts, like the Isle of Skye, as it is in towns like London. Secondly, the rise in atopic eczema is equally as startling as the rise in hay fever and asthma—and it is difficult to see how atmospheric pollution could be responsible for this.

## A change in our immunity

This may well be where important changes have occurred. In the developed world our immune systems no longer have to deal with infectious illnesses that were commonplace years ago. Improved housing, antibiotics, and vaccinations have all contributed. Could this mean that our immune systems switch their attention to allergy? It is certainly possible but as yet, we do not know. The dietary changes that characterize the move from rural to city life may also impair immune responses.

All these possibilities need exploring—and other ideas need to be put forward, for there is no doubt that in our broad understanding of asthma there is no more pressing issue than that of the rising prevalence.

## What can we conclude?

This bird's eye view of the geography of asthma has served to emphasize again the dual influences of external and inherited forces. Climatic and socio-economic circumstances cannot alone induce asthma in those not inherently predisposed to it. Equally, given an inherited tendency to asthma, the environment—whether this be in terms of exposure to allergens, adverse weather conditions, industrialization, or domestic circumstances—can play a role in either facilitating or suppressing the expression of asthma. Thus whether viewed in the individual or in whole communities, there is no escape from the conclusion that asthma is truly a multifactorial disorder. It is the summation of the effects of inheritance and environment that determines whether asthma will or will not be experienced. The addition of one further trigger factor, however minor it might be on its own, may be sufficient to bring the underlying tendency to asthma out in the open. Conversely what might be of itself a minor adjustment in environment or medical management, may be all that is required to convert a troublesome persistent asthma to a mild and occasional wheezing. The treatment of asthma is considered in the next few chapters but just before launching into that story, we need to make some comments on the question of asthma deaths.

## Death from asthma

It would not be surprising, asthma being as common as it is, that some people would die with asthma. But can death occur because of the asthma itself? The answer, sadly, is yes. The processes described earlier that are responsible for narrowing the airways—mucus, swelling, tightening of the muscle around the air passages can, if excessive in degree, completely block the airways, so making it impossible to breathe at all.

Individual doctors will witness an asthma death very rarely. When they do so, it leaves a lasting impression. It is often sudden and unexpected, and especially poignant, when it occurs in a young person. Only the rather impersonal methods of study of the epidemiologists can give us an overall picture of the size of the problem, and help us to find clues to the reasons why asthmatics occasionally die of their condition.

For England and Wales statistics are available from death certificates. For the most part the figures are fairly reliable, though from time to time there are changes in classification that make interpretation of the trends a bit of a problem. The bar chart shows total asthma deaths by year from 1959 to 1992.

For much of this century, the number dying from asthma had been

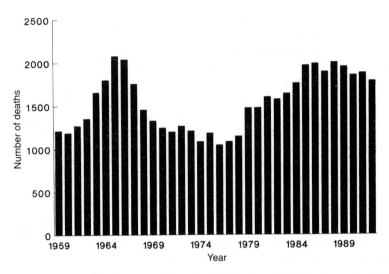

The numbers of asthmatics dying in England and Wales between 1959 and 1992.

extraordinarily stable: but in the 1960s and again in the 1980s there were notable deviations from this trend. The general stability seems particularly surprising when we consider the great advances that have been made in the treatment of asthma in the last forty years which we might have expected to improve the figures.

The upsurge in deaths in the 1960s was closely scrutinized. It occurred chiefly in young people and came at a time when pressurized aerosols for the relief of asthma were being marketed over the counter. As the sales went up, so did the deaths. When the association was pointed out, sales were stopped and the excess deaths ceased. How could a treatment that was so obviously beneficial be, at the same time, harmful? Two principal explanations were put forward. The first blamed side effects from the inhaled medicine, and the second postulated that the young asthmatics relied too heavily on these relieving inhalers. In an acute attack they became complacent and failed to seek medical advice until it was too late. We shall be talking about these inhaled medicines in more detail later (Chapter 11). Suffice it to say that a similar criticism against another relieving inhaler was made, in New Zealand, in the 1980s where they experienced a fourfold increase in asthma deaths over a period of four or five years.

In the UK there was a second increase in asthma deaths with the figures almost doubling between 1975 and 1985. This time the increase was slower and the relieving inhalers then in use were considered safer than those implicated in the earlier UK epidemic. The circumstances surrounding these deaths were different, and raised several issues beyond that of the possible dangers from the inhalers themselves.

The first point to note is that in this instance it was elderly people not the young who featured prominently. In the past, many elderly people with wheezy chests were thought to have 'bronchitis' of various sorts. Quite a number of these individuals would now be considered to have asthma. In other words, the observed increase in deaths may just have been a change of label.

But secondly, this rise in deaths came at a time when the prevalence of asthma was on the increase. More asthmatics will surely mean that a greater number of deaths could be expected. This is certainly true, providing the increase in numbers of asthmatics occurs equally across all grades of severity of asthma. The stickler here is that the number of deaths has increased in the elderly rather than in young people, whereas the increased numbers of asthmatics are most clearly documented in the young. Furthermore when we look at the number of people seeking attention for asthma, again it is amongst the young that admissions to hospital and consultations have been most obviously rising.

The failure of these two explanations has forced attention to be focused on how asthma is treated. The issues are, however, broader than just the medication and take into consideration how we look after asthmatics, what provisions are made for their care, what precautions are taken to keep them well and what measures can be adopted to avoid attacks, and especially to avoid deaths. The organization of care for asthmatics has certainly, at times, not been ideal, and the efforts put into helping asthmatics look after themselves in order to prevent trouble have left something to be desired. In any survey of asthma deaths, criticism of care provisions comes into the picture for at least some of the deaths. A detailed look at the management of asthma is, therefore, of vital importance. This follows in the next few chapters.

# Control of asthma

# 10 *An introduction to the treatment of asthma*

Over the seventeen years since the first edition of this book, there have been subtle but important changes in the treatment of asthma and of asthmatics which need spelling out before we can proceed to look in detail at the treatments currently available.

These changes involve shifts of emphasis rather than anything fundamentally new. The greatly increased understanding we now have of the nature of asthma has resulted in a shift in our use of medicines away from just relieving wheeze, in favour of preventing the wheeze occurring in the first place. But also our greater appreciation of the impact of asthma on everyday life has led to a shift in care, away from reliance on the doctor all the time, in favour of self-management and personal decision making, issues we shall pick up again in Chapter 14.

## A brief review of how asthma comes about

It would be helpful, at this stage, to recall some of the salient points of earlier chapters, which dealt with the mechanisms of asthma to see how present day treatments dovetail in with our improved knowledge. We can start from the observation that the symptoms of asthma are due to narrowing of the air passages within the lungs (p. 26). The narrowing is due to a combination of tightening (or spasm) of the muscle which spirals around the air passages, swelling of the walls of the air passages, and to mucus blocking them off. These three processes are all the result of inflammation (p. 67). The inflammation is caused by the presence of chemical messengers (mediators) and these mediators are themselves released from cells that are naturally present in the air passages, especially the mast cells (p.59), or from cells that crowd into the airways in asthma, particularly the eosinophils (p. 68). The final link in the chain asks what triggers these cells to release their mediators. Chapter 4 illustrated how allergy does this: exercise can also trigger mast cells to disrupt, and infection does so by mechanisms that are still not fully clear. So there is a sequence: triggers such as allergy cause cells to release mediators, which in turn cause inflammation which results in narrowing and blockage of the airways.

## Opportunities for treatment

Such a sequence presents many opportunities for tackling the asthmatic process. Perhaps an analogy will help. Along a route I regularly take, I find that I frequently knock my shin on an obstacle. There are four ways of dealing with the situation. Give my shin a rub and take a couple of aspirin to relieve the pain: wear a pad on my leg to protect my shin: avoid that route altogether: or take a pick axe and remove the obstacle. We can call these four approaches symptom relief, protection, avoidance, and cure.

An approach like this can be applied to asthma. You find that wheeze regularly occurs under certain circumstances. To take an inhaler that immediately relaxes tight airways is the first approach—symptom relief. To take regular treatment which dampens down your inflamed airways is the second approach. To never allow yourself to go near the cause of your wheezing is avoidance. Sadly there is, as yet, no pick axe to bring about a cure for asthma.

The move away from just relief towards prevention is achieved most commonly by the use of preventive medication. Protection, the word that fitted the obstacle analogy, is not conventionally used for this step in asthma treatment. Rather these medicines have become known as preventers. Even this word seems not entirely appropriate, both because there are other ways of preventing asthma and because these medicines have actions that are more active than the word prevention implies. Indeed they are anti-inflammatory and it has become increasingly clear that taking regular treatment to suppress inflammation is the best way of controlling asthma. Relief medications are then needed only rarely. And if precautions can be taken to avoid triggering asthma, control is further improved. We have not yet learnt how to stop people having asthma altogether. It is not a forlorn hope to imagine that one day this might be possible. Understanding the genetic basis of allergy or the unravelling of mechanisms which seem to perpetuate inflammation in the airways, may well lead to a true cure. But that is not available yet. Hopefully it is round the corner. Till then it is a matter of using the medicines and avoidance measures that we have currently available to their best possible advantage.

## Relief, prevention, or a combination of both

It would be a simple matter to understand the treatment of asthma, if certain medicines only gave relief and others were exclusively preventative. To a degree that is true. Those medicines, the bronchodilators, which open up (dilate) tightened air passages (bronchi) are the medicines which pre-eminently give relief. But these same remedies employed in different ways can be used as preventers, and we lose an important dimension in treatment if we only think of bronchodilators as a means of giving immediate relief from symptoms.

And what of the medicines that we call preventers. Both those in current use and others still experimental all in some way tackle the processes that make asthmatic airways inflamed and irritable. Thus they are all 'anti-inflammatory'. The best known of these treatments is steroids which, like other medicines in this category, have a powerful effect in dampening down inflammation. Yet, whilst steroids do not give immediate relief, they can be very useful in treating acute severe attacks of asthma. So they seem more than just preventers; they are active participants in treatment. However, because of the strong tradition for using the word 'preventer' for all these types of treatment, this is the convention adopted in the remaining chapters on the treatment of asthma. Other approaches to prevention that involve the avoidance of trigger factors also come up for consideration (Chapter 14).

## A look ahead

With this introduction in mind, we can now look in some detail at how asthma is treated and how it can be managed overall to produce a good quality of life free of symptoms and with you, the asthmatic, confident that you are in charge.

The sequence looks like this. First, the use of bronchodilators to give relief (Chapter 11): secondly the value of steroids and other medicines to tackle asthmatic inflammation (Chapter 12): thirdly we take a practical look at inhaler devices (Chapter 13): next, ways of avoiding asthma through environmental control (Chapter 14): then an overview of how asthma care is organized at different ages and in varying circumstances (Chapter 15): and finally a drawing together of some remaining issues to complete our picture of living with asthma (Chapter 16).

# 11  *Bronchodilators and the relief of symptoms*

•••••••••••••••••••••••••••••••••••••••••••••••

Success in the quick relief of the symptoms of asthma centres on the use of the bronchodilators, which 'open up' the narrowed airways by an action primarily on bronchial muscle. What sort of medicines are these and how do they work?

It will be recalled from Chapter 3 that when we prepare out bodies for activity we bring into play what is called the sympathetic nervous system. This quickens the pulse, increases the blood pressure, tenses the muscles, and opens up the bronchi of the lungs so that we can breathe more easily. As far as the lungs are concerned, this result is not directly achieved by nerves which supply the lungs but indirectly by a chemical messenger sent to all parts of the body from some small glands sitting on the top of the kidneys. These adrenal glands pour out into the bloodstream their messenger, adrenaline, when they are stimulated into activity by the sympathetic nervous system.

## The early history of bronchodilators

Adrenaline was discovered towards the end of the last century by an enterprising general practitioner, Dr Oliver. Sir Henry Dale eventually purified the chemical messenger, and the commercial development of adrenaline as a bronchodilator for asthma followed in the 1920s.

This was not by any means the beginning of bronchodilator therapy. A 4000-year-old Chinese herbal remedy, Ma Huang, a cough linctus, contained the first known bronchodilator, ephedrine. In Roman times, Pliny the elder recorded that ephedrine was taken in sweet wine, for the treatment of asthma. Thereafter it seems to have been forgotten till this century. In 1913 Japanese investigators isolated ephedrine and it was marketed there as 'Asthmatol'. Ephedrine was the first class of drug to possess properties which mimic the action of the sympathetic nerves and so are called sympathomimetic.

So, some seventy years ago physicians were in a position to pre-scribe two powerful bronchodilator drugs: adrenaline and ephedrine.

Adrenaline was prepared as a solution for injection and for inhalation. Ephedrine was prepared as a tablet. Adrenaline was the standby treatment for acute asthma for both doctors and patients over many years. Injected under the skin slowly, in small quantities it was a powerful remedy.

## Pharmaceutical developments

Attempts followed to manufacture in the laboratory compounds with similar properties to these naturally occurring substances. Of the many such compounds, one stood out as highly effective: this was isoprenaline. As an aerosol for inhalation, it established itself as a potent and very rapidly acting bronchodilator.

But adrenaline, ephedrine, and isoprenaline all have their problems. They not only relax bronchial smooth muscle but also stimulate all parts of the sympathetic nervous system. This means that the blood pressure rises, the pulse races, the head thumps, and the pupils constrict. Ephedrine also affects the bladder, and causes anxiety and excitement. If the adrenaline is injected into a vein rather than being absorbed from under the skin, the action on the heart can be dangerous. Thus a search went on for more selective agents.

It was discovered that the chemical messengers work by attaching themselves to certain specific sites—known as receptors—on the surface of the muscles, rather like a key fits into a lock. Not all the receptors on sympathetic muscles turn out to be the same. The two main types were named alpha and beta. Alpha receptors caused blood vessels to constrict. The beta receptors seemed to predominate in bronchial muscle and were also found in the heart.

Perhaps of even greater value than the division of receptors into alpha and beta divisions was the recognition that not all beta receptors were identical. Those in the heart were labelled, beta 1, those in the bronchi, beta 2. The great importance of this discovery lay, of course, in the potential for finding drugs that would work on the beta 2 receptors—relaxing the bronchi and so relieving the asthma—without having a stimulant action on the heart through the beta 1 receptors. Drugs which activate a receptor are called 'agonists', so the name given to this group of sympathomimetic bronchodilators, which are so important in asthma treatment, is the $\beta_2$-agonists.

## Currently available β-agonist bronchodilators

A daunting array has been produced. Apart from introducing selectivity of action on $\beta_2$ receptors, it has been the aim of the pharmaceutical chemists to prolong the effect of these drugs without losing the immediacy of relief that is so much coveted by the patient. A list of the $\beta_2$-agonist bronchodilators currently available is given opposite. Salbutamol remains the most frequently prescribed $\beta_2$ selective bronchodilator in the UK. Terbutaline is very similar to salbutamol, and is used extensively in Scandinavia. Like fenoterol, it has a somewhat longer duration of action than salbutamol.

Duration of action is most certainly a property that can be built into a $\beta_2$-agonist bronchodilator. Speed of onset of action is very similar for all of them, though after the initial boost there may be a slow build-up of effect for about an hour with longer-acting drugs. It is not very meaningful to talk about the relative strength of these various drugs. The degree of relief possible depends on many factors of which only a few are directly related to the drug itself. Any of the $\beta_2$-agonist bronchodilators can be given in a dose that will produce the maximum effect possible in a given person at a given time. The most potent reason for not giving a drug in maximum dose would be an unwanted side effect. With a non-selective drug such as isoprenaline, the side effect limiting its use would probably be a fast pulse rate or a rise in blood pressure. With the more selective agents, cardiac effects are much less but they can cause a distressing tremor of the hands.

Setting aside the properties of the drug itself, the degree of response likely to be produced with a bronchodilator depends to a large extent on the individual and his asthma. Some types of asthma, or some stages of asthma in an individual, are more responsive to treatment than others. In general, when the asthma is severe, a bronchodilator will seem to have little effect. Likewise if there is little or no obstruction, the potential for improvement is small and again there will appear to be little benefit gained from using a bronchodilator. It is in the very broad range of intermediate degrees of obstruction from mild to moderately severe that bronchodilators are most effective.

In looking at how effective a bronchodilator is, we must also discuss the question of how it is given. All bronchodilators are effective when injected. This is neither desirable nor practical for the everyday management of asthma. Injection can be important for β₂-agonist bronchodilators

| UK approved name | Tablets | Aerosols | Injections | UK trade names | Other names |
|---|---|---|---|---|---|
| Adrenaline | | • | • | Medihaler-epi (+Aus) | Epiphrine (US) Bronkaid (US) Asthmahaler (US) Epi-pen (US) |
| Bambuterol | • | | | Bambec | |
| Ephedrine | • | | | CAM | Fedrine (Aus) Neo-respin (US) |
| Fenoterol | | • | | Berotec (+Aus) | |
| Isoprenaline | • | • | | Medihaler-Iso | Isoproterenol (US) Isuprel (US) |
| Ocriprenaline | • | • | | Alupent (+Aus) | Metaproterenol (US) Metaprel Promeva (US) |
| Pirbuterol | | • | | Exirel | Maxair (US) |
| Reproterol | | • | | Bronchodil | |
| Rimiterol | | • | | Pulmadil | |
| Salbutamol | | • | • | Aerolin, Salbulin Ventolin (+Aus) Volmax (+US) | Albuterol (US) Proventil (US) |
| Salmeterol | | • | | Serevent (+US) | |
| Terbutaline | • | • | • | Bricanyl, Monovent (+Aus) | Brethine (US) Brethaire (US) |
| Tulobuterol | • | | | Brelomax, Respacal | |
| Bitolerol | | • | | | Tornalate (US) |

the treatment of acute severe asthma and that aspect will be considered later. Facilities for patients to inject themselves with adrenaline are rarely provided now, both because of the ease with which other routes can give relief and because of the potential dangers of the adrenaline. So for general use there are but two routes to consider—by mouth or by inhalation.

Powerful reasons exist for giving bronchodilators by inhalation. Chiefly it is dose and side effects that need to be considered. Tablets or syrups taken by mouth must rely on much larger quantities of the drug being absorbed from the stomach and intestines in order to make available an adequate quantity for the lungs. For salbutamol the smallest inhalation contains 100 micrograms of the drug: the smallest tablet contains 2 milligrams (or 2000 micrograms)—20 times the dose of the inhalation. Thus the potential for side effects will be many times greater with tablets than when using inhaler therapy. This fact is not significantly offset by the observation that there is a strong tendency for patients to take more puffs from their inhaler than recommended either by doctors or by the pharmaceutical companies. This is in striking contrast to the general attitude towards tablets. It is usual that fewer tablets are taken than the number recommended and almost never more.

## How and when to use bronchodilator inhalers?

There are basically three patterns: for symptoms as they arise, as a preventative, anticipating symptoms; and repeated use. Bronchodilators are primarily a means of giving symptomatic relief for episodic wheezing. The chest becomes tight during the night, a wheeze develops walking up a hill. A puff from a bronchodilator aerosol will bring instant relief. For patients with mild asthma which for the most part is causing them no symptoms, and for patients with more severe asthma maintained on other therapy but having intermittent and unexpected spasms of wheezing, the inhaler is the friend they need.

There are circumstances where the bronchodilator aerosol can be used as a preventative. The wheezing that is seen after exercise can be prevented in almost all asthmatics by the prior inhalation of a bronchodilator. Other potentially wheeze-provoking situations can also be anticipated. An asthmatic sensitive to dogs could well take a bronchodilator inhaler before an unavoidable visit to a dog-keeping household.

More difficulty has arisen when attempting to provide a preventative dose of bronchodilator to cover the small hours of the night, and especially the low point about dawn when asthma attacks can occur. For many years the only way of tackling this was with the large dose slow release tablets of a bronchodilator such as salbutamol, terbutaline, or an aminophylline type medicine (see page 145). However now that the long acting inhaled bronchodilators have become available (e.g. salmeterol) it looks as though many patients troubled by nocturnal asthma will be fully controlled on these safer inhaled bronchodilators.

When asthmatics need some sort of bronchodilator last thing at night, and then several doses during the day, they almost imperceptibly move from a situation when they are using their bronchodilators just for relief and prevention, to one where they are using them repeatedly during the day. Until quite recently it was thought very sensible to use bronchodilators regularly. A standard recommendation would have been two puffs four times a day. The idea was to keep up the obvious short term benefit over longer periods of time. In practice this didn't seem to be the case. Asthmatics taking a regular bronchodilator four times a day were observed carefully over several months. Surprisingly they seemed to do rather less well than when they took their bronchodilator only when they needed it. Most of them were not

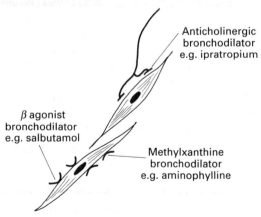

The actions of various bronchodilators.

taking any other asthma medications and it seems likely that this effect would be lessened or reversed if they also used a steroid inhaler. This sort of observation is one of those that is behind the change in emphasis towards the early regular use of preventative steroid aerosol treatment (see next chapter). Of course in more severe asthma, many asthmatics do use their bronchodilators on a regular basis every 4–6 hours, and certainly could not manage without them. The message here is that on no account should asthmatics rely on regular bronchodilators *alone*. If their asthma is that severe, they need preventative treatment as well.

## A different sort of bronchodilator

It was noted earlier (p. 49) that some nerves of the autonomic nervous system cause contraction of bronchial muscle: these are the cholinergic or parasympathetic nerves. Through the activity of these nerves the normal bronchial muscle is kept 'toned up'; without it, the smaller bronchi might simply collapse. Excessive activity in these nerves can cause chest tightness in asthmatics. Fortunately this can be blocked with the drug atropine, which is thus known as an anti-cholinergic.

Like ephedrine, atropine has a long history. It is extracted from the plant *Atropa belladonna*. The name has a lurid derivation. In Greek mythology Atropos was one of the three fates who cut with shears the web of life. Atropine has been used as a poison. Dilute extracts of the plant were at one time fashionable as eye drops to dilate the pupils, hence 'belladonna'. As a herbal remedy it has had an established place in the Indian subcontinent for over 4000 years. It was recommended that the leaves be smoked in a pipe till 'the chest, throat, and head become light, and the cough reduced'. Brought to this country through British Army physicians stationed in India in the last century, it has had a rather chequered history, falling in and out of favour. Renewed interest in atropine as a bronchodilator has arisen as a result of experiments which have shown that atropine can prevent some sorts of asthmatic wheezing.

An atropine effect is achieved today with the inhaled drugs ipratropium and oxitropium. Both are available as pressurized inhalers and there is a nebulizer solution of ipratropium. In practice, the benefits to be obtained from the use of these agents in asthma turn out to be limited. They will help some asthmatics but the sympathomimetic drugs have a similar and usually greater effect. This is in contrast to the effect obtained in patients with chronic bronchitis who also get narrowing of the airways. In such patients atropine-like drugs are at least as effective as the sympathomimetics in relaxing the obstruction, and sometimes more effective. In a given individual there is often a mixture of factors leading to airways obstruction. Cigarette smoking and infection lead to bronchitis; heredity and allergy lead to asthma. The more features of allergy that are detectable, the less will be the response to atropine. It is the allergic component to the airways narrowing that is resistant to the action of atropine in man. After the allergic component has been treated any residual airways narrowing will then respond to atropine.

## One more bronchodilator

One other group of medicines, known as the methylxanthines, can also open up asthmatic airways. These agents are closely related to the caffeine found in coffee and tea. Though caffeine itself has only a small effect on bronchial muscle, it does have the very useful stimulant action of many sympathomimetic drugs on the flagging brain. Legend has it that the stimulant action of coffee was discovered by an Arabian prior. Learning from the local shepherds that goats which had eaten berries from the cocoa plant gambolled and frisked all through the subsequent night, the prior copied them to help him maintain his vigil through long nights of prayer.

The drugs in this group best known to asthmatics are theophylline and aminophylline. Like adrenaline they are most dramatically effective when injected. Unlike adrenaline they may be given directly into a vein. They do have a stimulant action on the heart and must be injected slowly. Given in this way aminophylline was for a long time the preferred treatment for acute asthmatic attacks. It has now been superseded by the $\beta_2$-agonist bronchodilators such as salbutamol given by nebulizer (see p. 170).

Theophylline and aminophylline cannot be prepared in a form suitable for inhalation, so for more routine use they are taken by mouth. The pure drugs irritate the stomach: nausea and sickness are the results. So the pharmaceutical companies have tried to overcome this by changing the way in which these drugs are made into tablet form. Besides being more palatable, several preparations are now available in a slow-release form. As with the slow-release salbutamol they give benefit for 10–12 hours and so can be taken twice daily.

Methyl-xanthine bronchodilators.

| UK approved names | UK trade names | Other names |
|---|---|---|
| Aminophylline | Phyllocontin | |
| Choline Theophyllinate | Choledyl Sabidal | Brondekon (Aus) |
| Theophylline | Labophylline Lasma Nuelin Slo-phyllin Theo-dur Uniphyllin | Bronchodyl (US) Elixophyllin (US) Uni-dur (US) Uni-phy (US) |

So what is the place of theophylline, aminophylline, and similar drugs in relation to the selective $\beta_2$-agonist bronchodilators. They are a second line of defence. They seem to smooth out some of the sharp jags in the swinging asthmatic process. Taken before going to bed, the slow release tablets will often protect against bothersome early morning wheezing. During the day their influence can add to the effect of the inhaled bronchodilator rather than replacing it. But despite this many doctors find that the side effects, particularly on the stomach, produced by these drugs are not sufficient to outweigh the advantages they have, and prescribe them only sparingly.

One last word about these drugs introduces a totally different issue. Studies have shown that drugs like theophylline can modify lymphocyte immune responses in a way that could be beneficial to asthmatics. How valuable this approach will be, remains to be seen.

Mention needs to be made now of tablets which contain more than one bronchodilator. The only one now available is Franol. It contains the sympathomimetic, ephedrine, and theophylline. Mixtures such as these are frowned upon. It is especially important that the elderly be dissuaded from using preparations containing ephedrine because of the very adverse effects it can have on bladder emptying.

Bronchodilators represent an essential stepping stone in the therapy of bronchial asthma. They relieve the tightness and wheezing caused by narrowed airways. They can be used to anticipate situations likely to provoke asthma. Overwhelmingly the best way to deliver a bronchodilator is by the inhaled route. But though they give relief, and though they can afford some protection, their effects are short-lived. They appear to have no lasting influence on the underlying asthmatic process. For this we must turn to a consideration of medicines which protect asthmatic airways—the preventers.

# 12 *Steroids and the suppression of bronchial inflammation*

• • • • • • • • • • • • • • • • • • • • • • • • • • • • • • • • • • • • • • • • • • • • • • • • • •

The tightening of the asthmatic's airways that is so successfully, though temporarily, relieved with a bronchodilator, is a result of airways inflammation. Bronchodilators effectively relax the muscles that constrict the airways, but can't do much about the swelling of their walls or about the mucus that blocks them off. These, too, are the results of airway inflammation.

So a more comprehensive approach to dealing with the effects of asthma would be to tackle the inflammation itself, rather than only dealing with the tightened muscles. The best known and most effective way of doing this is with steroids, though other treatments do exist and exciting new approaches are on the horizon.

Despite over two decades of strikingly successful use of steroid inhalers as treatment in asthma, the legacy of fear left by the undisciplined use of steroid tablets in the 1950s and 60s means that any sort of steroid treatment in asthma can still be viewed with apprehension. So what are steroids and why are they so central to the modern management of asthma?

## A short history of steroids

The word steroid, in scientific terms, refers to a large group of substances having a common structure. In medical terms most steroids of interest are hormones. The sex hormones are steroids. So is the contraceptive pill. Unscrupulous athletes use androgenic steroids to artificially increase muscle strength. We are not concerned with any of these but with steroids which are made from the outer surface of the adrenal gland, the adrenal cortex. These are given the name corticosteroids. Corticosteroids are essential to life. Without them, as Addison first described in 1855, the body wastes away and the blood pressure cannot be maintained. Extracts of the adrenal cortex were first prepared during the 1930s and the individual steroids identified. Of most general interest are cortisone and the closely related hydrocortisone. The production of these hormones by the adrenal gland is under the direction of another hormone, adrenocorticotropic hormone (ACTH) secreted by the pituitary, a gland which nestles in the depths of the skull, underneath the brain.

Throughout the 1940s there was intense interest in discovering the natural role of adrenal corticosteroid hormones. Hans Selye pioneered the notion that they were concerned with the body's response to stress. Acting through the brain, stress causes an outpouring of ACTH, which in its turn stimulates corticosteroid output by the adrenal glands. Many illnesses, he pointed out, were accompanied by so-called non-specific symptoms which most physicians ignored; tiredness, listlessness, loss of appetite, and so forth. Selye argued that these symptoms arose because of maladaptation of the pituitary/adrenal system.

Complementary to this train of thought was the observation that during pregnancy when many steroid hormones are produced by the body, there is a general sense of well-being and patients with arthritis often experienced relief from their joint pains. Against this· background Hench tried giving cortisone to a patient with acute rheumatoid arthritis. The result was dramatic. The impact of this discovery on medicine can be gauged by noting that a year later, in 1950, Hench and the chemists who had isolated and purified cortisone received the Nobel prize for Medicine.

Soon cortisone was being tried in a wide variety of conditions with varying but often striking success. One of these conditions was asthma. It was very quickly evident that steroids would combat severe life-threatening attacks of asthma. Disappointing relapses then began to appear when the steroids were withdrawn, and before long it emerged that long-term maintenance treatment was essential in some patients. This policy brought with it the spectre of slowly progressive and potentially serious side effects, which caused something of a reaction against the use of steroids in the late 1960s. The pendulum has now swung back to a more sensible position, partly due to the skills learned from experience, but chiefly due to the introduction of steroids which can be given by inhalation.

## How do steroids work?

Surprisingly little is known about the way in which steroids produce their beneficial effects in asthma. Although this in no way limits their use as an effective treatment, it does represent a failure in understanding that could have important implications. Undoubtedly steroids are one of the most powerful of all anti-inflammatory drugs. Inflammation, it has been seen (Chapter 4), is a crucial feature of the processes which create asthma. Steroids control and reduce inflammation: and so they control and reduce the symptoms of asthma. Samples from the lining of the airways of asthmatics treated with steroids show far fewer mast cells and eosinophils (see Chapter 4). Because of this there are fewer of the unpleasant chemicals that perpetuate the asthmatic inflammation.

In a more practical sense it has been shown that steroids protect against allergy, not against immediate allergy but against the late reaction at 4–6 hours. Finally, though steroids are not bronchodilators, they do help bronchodilators to be more effective.

Not long after the introduction of the natural corticosteroids, which were extracted from the adrenal glands of animals, it became possible to manufacture corticosteroids in the laboratory. The aim, as so often in pharmaceutical research, has been to eliminate side effects and improve the beneficial effects. This has not been as successful with steroids as with some other drugs. The main achievement has been to make the manufactured steroids more powerful weight for weight than the natural corticosteroids. This has been accompanied by a slight emphasis in favour of the effects thought likely to be most beneficial in treating illnesses, and against some of the side effects.

## Inhaling steroids

Just as for the bronchodilators, the preferred route for giving steroids for asthma is by inhalation. An attempt to administer steroids directly to the lungs of asthmatics was made in the early days of corticosteroid manufacture. Unfortunately these steroids were absorbed into the body equally readily whether given by inhalation or swallowed. This meant that, as far as side effects were concerned, the inhalation route offered no advantage and therapeutically both routes were equally effective.

Research stimulated by the need for poorly absorbed steroids for skin conditions, resulted in the manufacture of steroids which could also be used by inhalation. Beclomethasone, budesonide, and now fluticasone are the most used inhaled steroids in asthma.

Steroid inhalers have transformed the management of asthma. They are the major preventative treatment in current use and are employed exclusively as a long-term maintenance therapy. In many asthmatics,

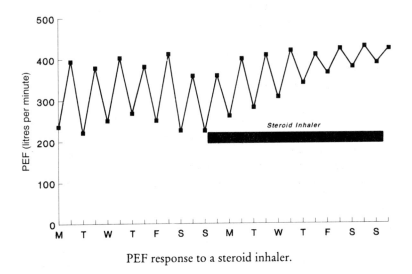

PEF response to a steroid inhaler.

steroid inhalers need to be given only twice daily, though sometimes three or four times daily is preferable. Because inhalers were first introduced for bronchodilators, there has been an unfortunate tendency for patients to regard the steroid inhalers as another way of obtaining quick relief. If they do, they will be disappointed. Steroid inhalers do not give immediate relief and their true worth only emerges with continuous use. For many asthmatics they are the very best preventative measure for keeping asthma under control. An effect can be noticed within a few days of starting therapy. If serial peak flow measurements are being made, it is often the loss of the 'morning dip' that is first seen. Then the overall level of peak flow gradually rises giving complete freedom from wheezing in the majority of patients in whom they are used. Once on steroid inhaler therapy, histamine is less likely to cause the asthmatic to wheeze, so is exercise, so are the challenges with allergens that cause late reactions.

Side effects have not been serious. Hoarseness is the commonest complaint. It is usually due to a chemical inflammation of the larynx. Sometimes there is an infection with a yeast-like fungus called *Candida*. The infection is usually evident in the back of the throat and on the palate where it causes the white patches that give it its common name, thrush. Thrush is somewhat less likely to occur if the mouth is rinsed with water after using a steroid inhaler, if the inhaler is taken twice daily rather than four times, or if a spacer device is used. *Candida* infection causes an unpleasant sore throat, and while it can be treated with anti-fungal drops or lozenges, it is the commonest reason for having to stop steroid inhalers. Steroids continually rubbed into the skin cause it to become thin and vulnerable to injury. Fortunately there is no evidence that the same problem occurs in the throat or bronchi. But sufficient steroid can be absorbed into the body with high doses of inhaled steroid to cause skin bruising and even some thinning of the bones.

## Steroid tablets

With the success of steroid inhalers, the role of steroid tablets has dwindled. However they are still needed for progressively deteriorating asthma and for severe asthma attacks. A single dose of prednisone will produce detectable relief in an asthmatic in about three hours though its maximum effect is not evident for about nine hours. In practice, a course of prednisone tablets rather than a single dose is used. In many attacks of asthma prednisone tablets starting at 30–40 mg a day are usual and maintained until a good effect has been produced. This is then followed by a lower dose, often for a similar period of time, to ensure maximum dampening down of the inflammatory process in the airways. Such a course is short, sharp, beneficial, and does not produce side effects. Indeed a course like this can be repeated several times a year if necessary without ill effect. If a longer course is required, generally when the attack is more severe, it may be initiated with an injection of hydrocortisone and may need to be continued for up to three or four weeks.

Patients who have required a course of prednisolone by mouth will need the beneficial effects of this treatment prolonged and maintained by continuing to take steroids in inhaler form.

In a small number of severe asthmatics, in spite of the use of steroid inhalers, or because for some reason they cannot be used, it is necessary to think in terms of regular daily prednisolone by mouth. What generally happens is that unacceptable wheeziness returns within a few days of stopping a course of prednisone or even before it has been stopped. Making the decision to institute long-term maintenance steroid therapy is not easy. Steroids have a bad, and not unjustified,

Steroid inhalers, tablets and injections used in the treatment of asthma

| UK approved names | Inhaler | Tablet | Injection | UK trade names | Other names |
|---|---|---|---|---|---|
| Beclomethasone diproprionate | ✓ | | | Aerobec<br>Becotide (+Aus)<br>Becodisks<br>Becloforte (+Aus) | Beclovent (US)<br>Vanceril (US) |
| Budesonide | ✓ | | | Pulmicort | |
| Fluticasone proprionate | ✓ | | | Flixotide | |
| Dexamethasone | (✓/US) | ✓ | ✓ | Decadron (+Aus) | Hexadrol (US)<br>Dalalone (US) |
| Hydrocortisone and cortisone | | ✓ | ✓ | Cortistab   Hydrocortistab<br>Cortisyl   Hydrocortone<br>Solu-cortef   Efcortelan | Cortone (US) Cortate (Aus)<br>Cortef (US + Aus) |
| Methyl-prednisolone | | ✓ | ✓ | Medrone<br>Depomedrone | Medralone (US)<br>Depomedrol (US)<br>Medrol (Aus)<br>Depomedrol (Aus) |
| Prednisone and prednisolone | | ✓ | ✓ | Precortisyl<br>Prednesol | Prednalone (US)<br>Hydeltrasole (US)<br>Deltasone (US) |
| Triamcinolone | (✓/US) | | ✓ | Kenalog<br>Ledercort | Azmacort (US)<br>Kenacort (US + Aus) |
| Flunisolide | (✓/US) | | | | Aerobid (US) |

record of causing ill health through side effects. A careful balance must be struck between intolerable disability due to the asthma and the possibility or even inevitability of side effects. Chronic asthmatics can often be kept in very good health on a dose of prednisone between 5 and 10 mg each day. At this level, even after many years, side effects are mostly not serious. Side effects become more likely if the dose is raised very much above 10 mg per day and can be lessened somewhat by taking the steroid on alternate days.

## Side effects from steroid tablets

Because there is, rightly, concern about the side effects of steroids, it is worth having some idea of the frequency with which they can be expected.

The most obvious unwanted effect of taking corticosteroids by mouth for any length of time is a gain in weight. This is partly attributable to stimulation of the appetite and partly to an interference with the way in which the body handles foodstuffs. Much of the weight gain is due to the laying down of fat, especially around the trunk and on the face, and it becomes obvious in about one-third of asthmatics taking continuous corticosteroids for more than a year. Some also show evidence of swelling of the ankles, suggesting the retention of fluid in the body. With fluid retention there is often a rise in blood pressure, though this likely in less than one in ten. Two other important side effects appear in about one-sixth of those asthmatics requiring continuous corticosteroids for more than a year—these are indigestion sufficient to lead to a definite stomach ulcer, and thinning of the bones sufficient to lead to a fracture. Few asthmatics require continuous steroids for this long. If courses are given intermittently, or if the dose is adjusted so that it can be taken every other day, then the frequency with which these more dramatic side effects is seen is much reduced.

Corticosteroid treatment interferes with certain internal defence mechanisms against infection and the stress of injury. A few asthmatics experience some change of mood on corticosteroid therapy. In the doses required by most, this is rarely serious and is more likely to be an elevation in mood rather than a depression. Thinning of the skin and easy bruising are common in the elderly requiring maintenance corticosteroids. In children the commonly seen weight gain is made rather more obvious by a retardation in height gain.

There is one additional long-term effect which is an inevitable consequence of continuous oral steroid therapy. This is the suppression of the adrenal glands' normal response to stress. Fortunately this does not occur with steroid inhalers in the doses generally required, though it can occur with higher doses totalling 2 mg of beclomethasone and more each day. In health, the adrenal glands naturally produce a quantity of cortisone equivalent to about 5–7 mg of prednisone a day. If prednisolone tablets are being taken each day, they are so equivalent to the natural hormone that the adrenals no longer need to manufacture their own cortisone. The amount taken is not, however, adequate for times of stress—the stress of a road accident, an operation, an infection, even an acute attack of asthma. Normally the adrenal glands would respond to these situations by pouring out more cortisone, but if their manufacturing processes have been suppressed for months on end because steroids have been taken, they cannot respond quickly enough to the demands placed on them. Indeed sometimes they cannot respond at all.

This problem has important implications when it comes to altering steroid doses. The natural history of asthma is such that there are times of life in a given individual when asthma is bothersome, and others when it is less so. Maintenance steroid therapy instituted in a time of severe asthma may later become unnecessary. But steroids cannot, must not, be stopped abruptly. If that happens, the adrenal glands will have insufficient cortisone reserves even for everyday life. Given time, they will recover. During this time the dose of steroid will need to be reduced very slowly, perhaps by as little as, for example, a 1 mg reduction in the total daily dose of prednisone each month. This very gradual tailing down will enable the stimulating hormone (ACTH), produced naturally by the pituitary gland in response to stress, to exert its control over the dormant adrenal cortex once more. It was thought at one time that injections of ACTH might hasten this process, but in fact this is not so.

If you are on corticosteroids, you should carry a 'Steroid Card' with you, which gives details of your treatment. You could also wear a Medic-Alert disc on a bracelet or neck chain. If you are unfortunate enough to be involved in an accident, if you need an operation, or if you develop certain acute illnesses, you may need more corticosteroid treatment than that necessary just to control your asthma. The attending doctor will know what to give by reference to your steroid card. Finally, never stop corticosteroid treatment abruptly. It is unwise to make sudden changes in any of the treatment used in asthma, but it can be positively dangerous suddenly to reduce drastically or stop corticosteroid treatment.

## Other attempts to block asthmatic responses

We have seen that once the allergic reaction has been triggered off, various chemicals are released which are either directly responsible for airways narrowing, or which attract into the airways cells which have damaging effects, particularly eosinophils.

One of the chemicals released from mast cells is histamine (see page 39). So it would seem logical to use antihistamines in treating asthma. These medications are widely effective in hay fever and allied allergic conditions of the nose, but they have been relatively unsuccessful in asthma. This is likely to be because histamine is only one of several mediators responsible for the asthmatic airway narrowing. The same fate may well befall other attempts to block individual mediators. Several drugs which antagonize the actions of the leucotrienes have been tested. They work in stylized laboratory settings, but seem unsuccessful in the day to day management of clinical asthma.

There is a growing awareness that one of the most important cells involved asthmatic inflammation is the lymphocyte. Lymphocytes grow wildly in certain sorts of leukaemia, and are instrumental in causing the body to reject tissue it recognizes as foreign. It is a short step then to use drugs found to be beneficial in leukaemia and transplantation, in asthma. They are powerful and potentially dangerous. They are used in intractable chronic asthma and in particular cyclosporin is showing some promise. Hopefully safer drugs will one day be produced following this principle.

## Intal and prophylaxis

Prophylaxis is a special form of preventative treatment. Taking anti-malarial prophylaxis when visiting the tropics works by killing off the malaria parasite the minute it enters the body. In asthma the idea is to interfere with the processes that start off the inflammation rather than just dampening it down by using steroids. The story of how this was first achieved is quite remarkable.

In the early 1960s the late Dr Roger Altounyan was investigating the properties of an Egyptian root from which an ancient remedy,

Khellin, had been derived. Khellin had been used for many years as a mild bronchodilator and for the relief of spasm in the bowel and kidney. Altounyan's contribution was to show that besides this property, Khellin contained a component which was not a bronchodilator but had anti-allergic properties. The purified compound disodium cromoglycate (DSCG) marketed as Intal proved to be the most powerful agent discovered in this research programme. It was shown to have very specific anti-allergic properties in immediate allergy. If given just before the inhalation of an allergen extract to which the subject was known to be sensitive, DSCG would protect against the airways narrowing normally to be expected.

It did not open up the airways as do the bronchodilators. Its effect waned after 4–5 hours, and it proved to have no effect if given after the challenge. It was not absorbed from the stomach and had to be given by inhalation. Taken four times a day as a prophylactic agent in a clinical setting, it often gave some improvement within days. Its maximal effect, however, was not evident for several weeks. Over this time it had an increasingly beneficial effect, reducing wheezing and chest tightness and lessening the need for bronchodilators and steroids.

Other interesting properties turned up on further study. DSCG afforded protection against exercise-induced asthma in about 60% of children. It reduced the sensitivity of the asthmatic to histamine; it improved the asthmatic's response to atropine. Laboratory studies suggest that all these activities are due to a stabilizing effect of DSCG on the mast cell. In the presence of DSCG the mast cell no longer breaks up when it meets an allergen and so no longer releases the damaging granules which go on to cause airway inflammation.

The patients who benefit most from DSCG are those who most clearly have atopic allergic asthma, and especially children. The response in adults is less predictable and there seems to be little or no protection against wheezing attacks precipitated by infection. In the atopic subject, DSCG is still the safest first choice after bronchodilators have failed to control symptoms. Side effects, apart from some irritation in the throat, are very uncommon.

DSCG does not dissolve easily in the propellants used for the pressurized aerosols and is best given as a dry powder (see page 166). Though it is available in a pressurized inhaler, each puff of aerosol only contains 5 mg compared with the 20 mg in each spincap. The pressurized inhaler therefore tends to be less effective. There

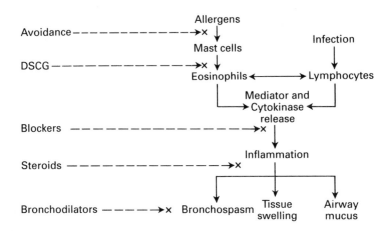

The mechanisms that cause airways narrowing showing where the various treatments for asthma act.

is also a nebulizer solution (20 mg per vial) which is excellent for very young children who cannot use other inhalers. For full effect, DSCG needs to be taken four times a day. It always requires a certain amount of discipline to remember the doses in the middle of the day.

DSCG has now been in widespread use for over twenty-five years and has made a very significant impact on both the management of asthma and research into understanding the intricate cascade of events that cause wheezing. A further prophylactic inhaler nedocromil is chemically dissimilar to Intal but has very much the same effect in asthmatics, protecting against allergen and exercise challenges and building up its beneficial effect slowly over several weeks. It has a bitter taste partly masked in the mint flavoured preparation. It is suggested that nedocromil need only be taken twice daily at a dose of two puffs (4 mg) each time. It may well be more effective taken three times a day and most adults will need 12–16 mg a day.

The various treatments described in this and the previous chapter fit into a sequence that runs parallel to the sequence of events that we believe to be responsible for the evolution of asthma. Though the list looks quite impressive, not all treatments are as effective as we would like and some have definite side effects. Medicines will only live up to their potential if we use them properly. So we now need to consider delivery devices specially designed for inhaled asthma medications.

# 13 *Practical issues in asthma treatment*

• • • • • • • • • • • • • • • • • • • • • • • • • • • • • • • • • • • • • • • • • • •

Having now seen how it is believed the various medicines for asthma work to control symptoms and improve lung function, we can now tackle important practical issues concerning how and in whom the medicines described are actually used. This chapter will give details of the ever changing range of inhaler devices available and illustrate how treatments can be used to best advantage at different ages.

## Inhalers, spacers, nebulizers . . . what are they?

Undoubtedly the most important reason for inhaling medicines in asthma is to deliver the treatment directly to the part of the body that needs it. Inhaling medication has two closely related advantages:

• A given improvement in the asthma can be achieved with a much smaller dose of inhaled medicine than that required in a tablet. The difference is quite large, of the order of tenfold.

• As a consequence of this smaller dose, there is much less chance of causing unwanted side effects.

In addition, there are a few asthma medications, such as DSCG, which are not effectively absorbed by mouth and so must be given by inhalation. On the other hand, some are too irritant to be inhaled and must be given by mouth, for example aminophylline.

Though the inhaler route has obvious advantages, not everyone finds it easy to use an inhaler. The very young, the elderly, the handicapped, or the just plain ham-fisted can find it difficult to set up inhaler devices or coordinate their breathing with triggering the device. Because of the importance of using the inhaled route and to help cater for everyone's needs, a large variety of devices have been manufactured. Despite this there are in fact only two ways in which medication can be prepared for inhalation. The first is to dissolve the medicine in a solution from which an aerosol (that is a mist of tiny particles) can be generated and then breathed in. And the second is to put the medicine into a powder which is pulled into the lungs by taking a sharp breath in. Much thought and technical sophistication have gone into making aerosols reliable, and into making powder devices user friendly, but at the end of the day there are just these two underlying principles that govern the production of inhalable medicines.

## Aerosol inhalers

### *Metered dose (pressurized) inhalers*

All asthma medications which can be inhaled are available in this form. The drug is dissolved in a mixture of organic solvents and sealed under pressure in a small canister. A jet of drug of measured size is released by pressing the canister into its plastic casing. To inhale the drug, the canister must be triggered just as a full breath in is being taken. Detailed instructions should be included in every pack of a pressurized inhaler you receive.

Errors in the use of these inhalers greatly reduce the effectiveness of the medication; but they are common. Most concern the timing of the firing of the canister. This should be done just after beginning to breathe in, not before, nor late in the breath. Breathing in should be from the end of a shallow breath out: it is not necessary to forcibly empty the lungs first. The breath in should be smooth and quite

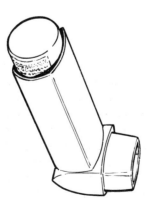

A pressurized aerosol inhaler.

slow, not a sudden jerk. It must be full and held for five to ten seconds.

---

### How to use a metered dose inhaler

1. Remove the cap and shake the inhaler
2. Breathe out gently
3. Put the mouthpiece in your mouth
4. Breathe in fully, not fast but not too slowly either
5. Immediately after beginning the breath in, press the canister to fire the inhaler
6. Hold the breath for about 10 seconds, then breathe out
7. Wait about 30 seconds before taking another inhalation

---

A question often asked is whether to take the breath in with the mouth open or the lips closed around the inhaler. It doesn't really matter, providing you are breathing in correctly. If you don't succeed in getting the medicine down, you will see it swirling around in your mouth, if you have your mouth open, or escaping up the gap between the canister and its casing, if you close your lips around the mouthpiece.

After holding the breath in, the chest is allowed to relax so that normal breathing can be resumed. If a second or subsequent inhalation is required, there is a specified waiting time, usually thirty seconds. This is not to allow you to get your breath back, but to allow the valve on the inhaler to recover, so that it delivers the correct amount of medication. Never press the canister more than once for a single breath.

Shaking the canister before you start mixes the medicine and the propellant together and also gives you some idea of whether it is full or empty. If you are concerned about the amount left in the canister, a useful tip is to drop it in a bowl of water. A full canister will sink: an empty one will float: and a partly full one will settle somewhere in between.

Currently the solvent in pressurized inhalers is a mixture of CFCs. Because of concern about the effect of CFCs on the ozone layer, their use, even in medications, began to be phased out during 1995. For the most part the design of the inhalers will alter very little, but hopefully the planet will be better off for the change.

Even with careful instruction and practice, these pressurized inhalers are quite difficult to use effectively. Fortunately, there are plenty of ways in which they can be adapted for easier use.

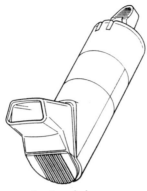

An Autohaler.

## The autohaler

This has the appearance of a completely encased pressurized aerosol. On the top there is a lever. When the lever is set, the gentle force of a breath in with the lips over the mouthpiece is enough to activate a trigger which opens the canister valve and fires the medicine into the mouth. This device, therefore, overcomes the problems of coordination, and gives good delivery to the lungs. Some people find that the sudden jet of medicine makes them briefly or even completely stop breathing in: in this case, the medicine is lost in the mouth.

The autohaler is available for salbutamol, beclomethasone, sodium cromoglycate, and oxitropium.

### Spacer devices

The sudden jet of medication on the back of the throat produced by the pressurized aerosols has two disadvantages. As noted above, it may interrupt the breath in. It does this through the cooling effect of the propellant as it evaporates on the back of the throat. But also it deposits quite a lot of medicine forcibly on the throat. This doesn't seem to matter much with the bronchodilators but there are problems with the steroids aerosols. With these the throat can become dry and sore, infection is encouraged (especially thrush, see p. 151) and the voice can become hoarse.

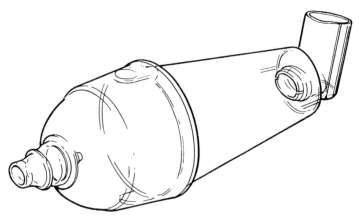

A large spacer (the Nebuhaler).

A clever solution to these problems was devised by Astra Pharmaceuticals. They noted that the puff from their inhaler came out about 20 cm and reached a diameter of about 8 cm. So they made a plastic container which would just envelop this cloud of medication. The device is called a Nebuhaler and is available for their products Pulmicort (budesonide) and Bricanyl (terbutaline). A similar device, the Volumatic, followed for the Allen & Hanbury's inhalers and there are now several others.

---

**How to use a spacer device, e.g. Volumatic**

1. Remove the cap, shake the inhaler, and insert into the end of the spacer
2. Put the mouthpiece in your mouth
3. Press the canister once to fire the inhaler
4. Take a deep, slow breath in
5. Hold the breath for about 10 seconds, then breathe out through the mouthpiece
6. Take a second breath in but do not fire the inhaler this time
7. Wait about 30 seconds before a second dose is taken

---

Once puffed into the spacer, the propellant in the mixture evaporates leaving tiny particles of the medication suspended in the air in the

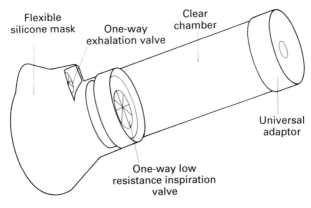

Flexible silicone mask
One-way exhalation valve
Clear chamber
Universal adaptor
One-way low resistance inspiration valve

The Aero chamber, a spacer suitable for young children.

spacer. They remain suspended for about five seconds, during which time they can be breathed in. The rule about using only one puff at a time from a metered dose inhaler still applies when using the spacer. A thirty second wait between inhalations is still required. For adults and older children the lips should make a good seal round the mouthpiece. For infants and young children it is better to use a spacer with a face mask.

There is some discussion concerning the best way to use these large spacers. If it is a question of using them for regular doses of a preventive (steroid) inhaler, then the breath in from the spacer should be full, deep, and held for at least five seconds. However, spacers are also useful for acutely wheezy asthmatics who need several puffs of a bronchodilator. They are too distressed to hold a breath in, and should be allowed to breathe in and out of the spacer in the way most comfortable for them.

The main problem with large spacers is their size. Though they pull apart to give two halves, this helps very little. However, since their main use is with the steroid inhalers which are generally taken twice a day, they usually do not need to be carried about.

Smaller collapsible spacers are an attempt to gain the advantages of the spacer device in a smaller, more easily portable way. They are not so successful and it is probably better to use the large spacer or turn to some other alternative.

Asthmatics with weak or arthritic hands may find it too much of an effort to press down the canister of the pressurized inhaler even though they may have no problems with coordination. For Allen and Hanbury's inhalers this problem can be overcome by using a Haleraid, which is suitable whether the inhaler is used alone or with a spacer device.

## Dry powder inhalers

An entirely different approach to the difficulties with pressurized aerosols is the dry powder inhaler. There is no propellant and so no concern over CFCs and the ozone layer. There is no automatic activation. The powder is inhaled by a forced breath in, almost a sucking action. The first dry powder inhaler—the Spinhaler was invented for use with Intal. The powder is in a capsule which is punctured when it is inside the Spinhaler. Sucking in from the inhaler then whirls up the medication into a cloud which is breathed in.

There are several further types of dry powder inhaler available. The Rotahaler takes capsules or Rotacaps of salbutamol (Ventolin) and beclomethasone (Becotide). They are broken open inside the device by rotating the mouthpiece on the body of the Rotahaler. The Diskhaler (for Ventolin, Serevent, Becotide, and Flixotide) houses a disc with up to eight blisters in it which can be punctured with a projection

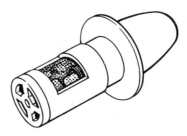

The Spinhaler.

## How to use the Spinhaler

1. Hold the Spinhaler upright with the mouthpiece pointing down and unscrew the grey casing
2. Put *coloured* end of spincap *into cup* of propeller
3. Screw the two parts together and move grey sleeve up and down at least twice to pierce the spincap
4. Breathe out gently, tilt the head back, put Spinhaler into the mouth and breathe in quickly and deeply
5. Remove Spinhaler from the mouth and hold breath for about 10 seconds

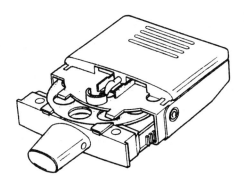

The Diskhaler.

## How to use the diskhaler

1. Remove the cap
2. To prepare the diskhaler for use, pull out the white tray, squeezing its sides so that it comes out of its shell
3. Put in a new circle of blisters with the numbers uppermost, then push the tray back
4. To use, hold the inhaler level and lift up the lid so that the projecting spike pierces the blister containing the medicine; close the lid
5. Then breathe out gently, and take a sucking breath in and hold for 10 seconds as for other dry powder inhalers
6. To prepare for the next dose pull the tray out so that the disc twists round; do no press the sides unless you want to change the whole disc

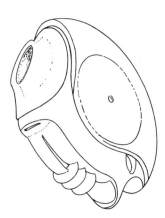

The Accuhaler.

fixed into the Diskhaler. The Turbohaler contains a reservoir of two hundred doses of powdered medication of Astra's products terbutaline (Bricanyl) and budesonide (Pulmicort). Each new dose is made available by twisting the bottom of the inhaler. Other multiple dose dry powder inhalers are the Aerohaler for ipratropium and oxitropium and the Actuhaler (for Ventolin, Serevent, and Flixotide).

Dry powder inhalers need to be kept in conditions where there is very little damp to avoid the particles of powder clogging together. Modern devices have proved very effective but have the disadvantage of depositing quite a proportion of the dose on the inside of the mouth.

### Which device?

What determines the choice of device? Because it is simple to operate, and cheap, metered dose inhalers are usually prescribed first for older children and adults. With careful tuition and regular checking, many asthmatics use these devices perfectly satisfactorily. However, for those who have problems using these aerosols, another device will need to be tried. If the inhaler only needs to be used at home, then the spacer devices are best. The dry powder inhalers are easy to use and more convenient when treatment has to be carried around. The powder sometimes causes coughing and the particles may stick on the mouth

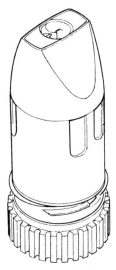

The Turbohaler.

## How to use the turbohaler

1. Unscrew and lift off the white cover. Hold the Turbohaler upright and twist grip clockwise as far as it will go and then back anti-clockwise
2. Breathe out gently, put mouthpiece between the lips and breathe in as deeply as possible
3. Remover Turbohaler from the mouth and hold breath for about 10 seconds

and throat. If this happens, it is back to the spacer device, though the conspicuous size of the larger spacers makes them embarrassing to use in public.

It must be emphasized that for everyone using inhalers and for everyone who has an interest in asthmatics who use inhalers, diligence in the proper use of them is absolutely vital. If you are asthmatic, check your own use of the inhaler that you have, particularly if it is the metered dose inhaler. Watch yourself in a mirror. Make sure that the inhaled medicine really is going down into your chest and read the instructions again if you are not sure. If you are the parent or carer of an asthmatic, make sure that your child or relative is following the instructions carefully. All asthmatics attending clinics should have their inhaler technique checked. One of the commonest reasons for a failure of medical treatment to be effective is that it's just not being taken properly.

### And what of nebulizers?

A further method of delivering inhaled medication is by nebulizer. It is basically another device which converts a solution of medicine

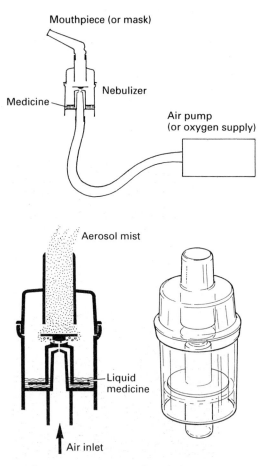

The component parts of a nebulizing system.

into an aerosol. This is breathed in via a mask or mouthpiece. The nebulizer unit, which is cheap, plastic, and disposable, must be driven by compressed air, usually from a robust, safe but portable electric compressor unit. These are quite expensive (£70–£100) but if well cared for and serviced, will last for several years, and a number of patients with asthma now have one (including Dr Storr as he describes in the introduction to this book).

The solutions available for use in nebulizers contain much larger doses of medicine than conventional inhalers particularly for the bronchodilator. This takes away the customary advantage of using inhalers, namely that by comparison with tablets, the dose is normally much smaller. However, in some situations, as we shall see later, larger doses of inhaled medicine are needed and this is where the nebulizers have such an advantage. The size and complexity of the nebulizer unit and compressor means that it is conspicuous and can be inconvenient to use outside the home, but for situations where the

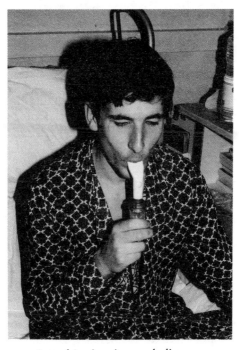

An asthmatic using a nebulizer.

large dose that the nebulizer can deliver is essential, the nebulizer can be life-saving.

Most compressors for nebulizers run on either mains electricity or, with a transformer, from a 12 volt car battery (using a lead that plugs into the cigarette lighter socket!). There is an alternative type of nebulizer unit, the ultrasonic nebulizer, which uses sound waves to shake up the solution of medicine into a vapour. It is more expensive and doesn't give quite such a reliable size of particle in the vapour, but it is smaller and can be battery driven.

## Combining treatment and device to best advantage

A look back over the last two chapters and the first part of this, reveals a wide range of treatments and an array of inhaler devices. It might at first sight seem almost impossible to weave these together to form a coherent way of treating different individuals with asthma. The ways in which they are used, however, form a relatively simple sequence.

The first treatment likely to be given to an asthmatic is a bronchodilator aerosol. This alone can be sufficient for mild intermittent asthma. If a bronchodilator is needed daily, or especially nightly, no time should be wasted before starting a preventative inhaler, a steroid, or DSCG. The dose and frequency are adjusted to bring the asthma under control. Failure to prevent nocturnal awakening, or to suppress daytime wheeze or shortness of breath, signifies the need to increase therapy. This means more steroid aerosol or adding in a longer acting or different type of bronchodilator. At every step inhaler technique and device used should be checked to ensure that the inhaled medicines are used to best advantage. The sharp attack associated with heavy exposure to allergens, a chest infection, or a slow build up of symptoms can be tackled with a short course of oral steroids.

Depending on the way the asthma presents, whether mildly and almost insidiously, or suddenly and severely, the first aim in treatment is to gain control of symptoms with whatever step or level of treatment is appropriate. After that the treatment can be reduced or altered to an optimum that maintains control and avoids side effects.

This pattern of using treatment to meet the demands of different degrees of asthma has become so much a habit that it has been set down in guidelines for the treatment of this condition.

A planned approach to treatment that pools the experience of experts in the field has much to recommend it. A consensus approach to guidelines helps the less experienced to choose treatments which the best available evidence suggests are sensible and effective. A set of guidelines for children was first put forward in the late 1980s. In the UK representatives of the British Thoracic Society, the National Asthma Campaign, and the Royal College of Physicians drew up guidelines for adults with asthma in 1991. These tackled both acute and persistent asthma and have now been updated twice, taking on board the views and experience of family doctors, paediatricians, and doctors who run hospital emergency departments. Similar guidelines have been produced in the USA, Canada, Australia, New Zealand, and elsewhere and important steps have been taken to produce internationally agreed guidelines.

## Adapting the treatment to suit different ages

### Infants and young children

It only takes a small amount of mucus or swelling of the lining of the airways to drastically narrow or shut off completely the tiny airways of young children. Most wheezy attacks in the first year or two of life are triggered by viral infection. Since there are no effective anti-viral drugs, the aim must be to clear the secretions and tackle the inflammation. A warm moist atmosphere and plenty of fluids by mouth will help keep the secretions liquid. Young children swallow their sputum rather than coughing it out—and this is the reason they often vomit with these infections.

Though not always very effective in young children, bronchodilators, both salbutamol and ipratropium are usually tried. A nebulizer or a spacer with a face mask make suitable delivery devices. It may be a little upsetting to press the mask down on the child's face but delivery of the medicine is more reliable this way. A distressed child with a serious attack requiring admission to hospital will benefit from inhaled steroids and may need oxygen.

### The pre-school child

Intermittent attacks may now have occurred sufficiently often to make it clear that the child has asthma. Even if allergic triggering of attacks is not necessarily obvious, the house dust mite and, a little later, household pets, are very often the underlying cause. For this reason, it is both advisable and sensible to start inhaled DSCG on a regular basis, again using either a nebulizer or a spacer with a pressurized inhaler. By the school years most children should be able to use a dry powder inhaler or an autohaler.

## School children

Bronchodilator inhalers are used on an 'as required' basis. Asthma during the night has conventionally been tackled with a syrup of salbutamol or theophylline, but salmeterol is coming into use for children as well as adults.

If DSCG has been effective and controls symptoms, its use should be continued. It has a place, too, as a prophylactic before exercise. Bronchodilators taken just before games are, however, more effective in preventing exercise-induced asthma.

Many children, by the school years, will have switched from DSCG to low dose steroid aerosols because of loss of control. It is not wise to persevere with treatment that fails to prevent nocturnal awakening, leaving the child listless and still wheezy in the day. The rewards of steroid aerosols in these children are enormous. They should be given twice daily, preferably with a spacer and pressurized aerosol.

Are there dangers? The chief concern has been over failure to grow. In fact careful analysis shows that uncontrolled asthma contributes more to growth retardation than do steroid aerosols.

A minority of children have sufficiently severe attacks to warrant oral prednisolone. Here growth retardation is more likely and must be balanced against the benefits from the treatment, and the disadvantages of living with uncontrolled asthma.

## The teenage years

Youngsters who still have troublesome asthma in the teens are likely to have had severe asthma in childhood. How they cope with the social demands of growing up with asthma will vary enormously. Those who have accepted the necessity for regular treatment will hopefully have relegated taking their inhalers into a routine habit. Those who rebel are likely to resent their disease and its management as much as they do other restrictions on their expanding lifestyle. Simplicity in treatment regimens is essential. A twice daily steroid aerosol with or without a long acting bronchodilator, and relief use of a short acting bronchodilator is usually practical. For those who choose to rely on their relief inhaler alone, the combined inhalers of a bronchodilator with either a steroid or DSCG should not be despised. Dry powder inhalers are usually less obtrusive than other devices (especially spacers), and some are now imaginatively packaged in a 'trendy' design. As with other chronic illnesses in teenagers, tact, consideration, and time are needed to pull young asthmatics through until maturity takes over.

## Adults

The planned approach described earlier is ideal for the adult patient with newly diagnosed asthma or asthma that has returned after some years of remission. The recommendations allow a level of treatment to be chosen that achieves control of symptoms and best possible lung function, whilst acknowledging the constraints that side effects may impose.

There are still areas of contention. Though steroid aerosols are generally started in a low dose (beclomethasone 800 μg daily or less), some advocate starting higher and reducing the dose quite quickly to the lowest level that sustains control. The choices after low dose steroids are multiple. Good evidence supports adding a long acting inhaled beta$_2$ agonist bronchodilator (e.g. salmeterol) rather than increasing the dose of inhaled steroid. Studies of other combinations are less convincing or unavailable, for example adding an anticholinergic or a theophylline-type oral bronchodilator. Little work is available to indicate whether a certain choice is better for a certain type of asthmatic or whether this is irrelevant.

In adults who need oral prednisolone every effort should be made to use the lowest acceptable dose. Alternate day treatment is often possible. Protection for thinning bones is wise in women after the menopause.

## The elderly

Similar principles underlie the choice of medication. Particular care is needed in choosing a suitable type of inhaler. Loss of muscular coordination or arthritic weakness make the use of pressurized aerosols a real problem. Some dry powder inhalers are very fiddly to load, and nearly all require good vision. Patient experimentation and instruction is needed to ensure inhaler treatment is optimally used. The opt out of using tablets, whilst in some ways attractive, should be resisted. Most have side effects of some sort, and these can be more dangerous in the elderly than in younger adults.

Now that we have seen how the medicines and devices available for asthma can be used, it is important to see how medication fits in with other aspects of the management of asthmatics. These include a variety of issues one of the most topical being the question of whether asthma can be prevented, we can then look at how care is organized for asthmatics and finally ask what it is like to live with asthma.

# Care and caring

# 14 *Can asthma be prevented?*

However effective the treatment of asthma may be, it would be better in the eyes of many of us if asthma could be prevented without resort to drug treatment. This chapter is chiefly devoted to asking what can be done to modify the environment in such a way that asthma is no longer provoked, but there has always been the hope that it might be possible to modify an individual's response, particularly to allergy, so that asthma does not develop despite provocation.

## Environmental control

The irritable airways of the asthmatic are influenced by a variety of triggers. Control can be exercised over some of these. Environmental temperature changes, fumes, fog, and similar irritants can be avoided up to a point. Infections can be reduced by taking evasive action. Psychological stresses may be amenable to resolution. But the possibilities for environmental control are focused most sharply on the question of allergens.

### *House dust mite control*

More effort has been put into reducing the dust load in the homes of those with dust mite allergy than any other form of environmental allergen control. Since the mite congregates wherever there are warm, humid conditions and human skin scales, it will predominate in bedrooms, in cushions, on carpets. Rigorous routines have been devised—vacuuming the mattress, especially under the buttons and piping, every other day; keeping the bedroom dry; wiping all flat surfaces with a damp cloth at least once a week. The bedclothes were to be shaken outside, whenever possible, and washed frequently. It was recommended that feather pillows, eiderdowns, and woollen blankets be replaced by others of synthetic material and carpets and heavy textured curtains avoided.

Was it all worthwhile? In individual instances parents and doctors have been convinced that dust control has made a significant difference to asthmatic symptoms. Disappointingly, comparisons of the progress of one group of children in whose homes dust control along these lines has been carried out, with another group where no such measures had been adopted, revealed few differences. If house dust mite sensitivity is such an important feature in childhood asthma, why have the results of dust control been so unimpressive? Perhaps chiefly because control did not reduce the mite load to sufficiently low proportions.

This view is supported by an interesting experiment in which a small group of asthmatic adults with dust mite allergy, slept every night for several months in a dust-free hospital unit. Though it took some weeks for any effect to become apparent, their symptoms did gradually improve and their airways became less irritable. So the possibility presented itself that if better methods of control could be devised, success might be achieved. This principle has been taken up in Denmark where houses have been designed and built with the specific aim of reducing the dust mite load. This is hardly practical on a widespread scale though reducing the temperature and increasing the ventilation are two alterations that can be adopted in any home. Beyond this, three new approaches are being evaluated: more efficient vacuum cleaners: mattress covers: and chemicals that kill off the dust mite (technically called acaracides).

The conventional domestic vacuum cleaner certainly sucks up dust from our carpets, but whilst the large particles are retained in the bag, a myriad of tiny particles, including the offending dust mite, are shot out into the room. Powerful, though expensive, vacuum cleaners are now fitted with much more efficient filters, reducing the load of dust that gets into the room by up to 90%. In one recent study, the cleaner manufactured by Voerwerk did especially well.

Covers have been suggested for many years as a means of containing the dust mite. Heavy duty plastic works, but sleeping on a mattress covered with that, can be unpleasant. Recent developments in this field have led to the marketing of a material that 'breathes'. The pores in it are just sufficient to let water vapour pass in and out, but not dust mites. Mattress covers are now commercially available under the brand name Intervent through Boots.

And so to acaracides. Chemicals certainly exist which kill off the dust mite. They still leave behind particles of mite which can be allergenic and not a few people have reservations about spraying their bedding and homes with powerful chemicals.

So where do we stand in relation to dust mite control? There is no doubt that these new techniques reduce the measured dust mite load in the air of the house. Do they also lessen the amount of asthma suffered by those allergic to the dust mite? This is much less well documented, but it seems likely that it will be so if the dust load is consistently reduced to very low levels. A contentious issue has been exactly how low and where the measurements of level should be made. Most studies have used samples of dust sucked up with a vacuum cleaner from carpets or the surface of mattresses. It has been argued quite sensibly that it would be more relevant to sample the air we breathe. This is now being done and the work suggests that previous recommendations gave 'safe' levels of dust that are too high. It is also showing that dust mite particles are not so readily released into the air from carpets made of synthetic fibres (as opposed to wool).

Even when skin testing and bronchial provocation suggest house dust mite allergy to be important, there may, in fact, be many other triggers that set off an individual's asthma. The loss of one trigger might not make a detectable difference to the overall pattern and frequency of asthmatic episodes. There is a suggestion too that the time in our lives that we first encounter an allergen, like the dust mite, may be very important. It is possible that in the first few months of life, even the first few weeks, even, it seems, in the womb, predisposed individuals may be unduly susceptible to the development of allergies. If this turns out to be true, it will make environmental control a much more acceptable strategy, since it may be required only for a limited time.

## Cats, dogs, and other pets

After the dust mite, the next most common household allergy is to pets. Doctors are often asked, 'Should the family cat, dog, guinea-pig, or whatever be sacrificed?' In the very few instances where an animal allergy is the only cause for asthma, the answer is clear enough. Often, as with the dust mite, it is only one allergy amongst many.

The importance of some animals is easy to assess. Cats are a good example. The cat allergen is on the animal's skin, fur, and present in its saliva. It is a very small particle and a powerful allergen. The moment the cat walks into the room, susceptible people will start to sneeze or wheeze. Removing the cat is obviously the prevention measure of choice but, if pussy is too precious, it helps greatly if it can be washed thoroughly each week, though it doesn't do much for the cat's dignity. This combined with good room cleaning, ventilation, and minimal carpeting and upholstery, can reduce the allergen load drastically. Testing this approach with other household pets might be equally successful, but if rodents, especially rats, are your penchant, then it needs to be remembered that a major allergy is to the animal's urine.

## The house itself

More serious questions are raised when general household conditions seem to be implicated in allergy. Should the asthmatic consider moving house? In only a few instances will the answer be 'yes'. Old and damp houses near rivers do harbour more house dust mites and moulds; dry, centrally heated houses and houses at high altitude, do not.

Indoor pollution is seldom a problem except for that produced by smoking. The adverse effects on the health of asthmatics of both active and passive smoking cannot be over emphasized. The question of gas cookers has also been referred to earlier. The message for prevention is obvious.

## Atmospheric pollution

The chances of asthmatics avoiding allergens, such as pollens, present in the outdoor environment are limited. Staying indoors on hot, windy summer days could be an advantage, but is restricting, and masks are of no value. Helmets with a power driven air filter can be a conspicuous but effective way of breathing clean air in hazardous working conditions. The concern expressed about urban atmospheric pollution from cars and factories is at a personal level just as difficult to translate into preventive action, but, at the political level, the situation could well be different. The tragic effects of the pea-souper smogs of the earlier years of this century directly led to the clean air acts which have transformed the outlook in respiratory disease in the last few decades. Now that interactions between environmental pollutants and allergy (see Chapter 8) are being identified, a further thrust to clean up the environment could well have long lasting benefits for asthmatics. Your MP is the entry point to this form of prevention.

## Occupational allergens

The prevention message from occupational asthma is almost too obvious to be stated. The discovery of a specific agent only produced in specific circumstances in a specified industry is a source of excitement, not only for what it can teach us about the inception and perpetuation of asthma, but also because it presents unique opportunities in prevention. It is not always easy to suggest changes in industrial practice that will eliminate the source of asthma in that setting, but it is nearly always possible to do something to make working conditions less hazardous.

The Health and Safety Executive takes the issue of occupational asthma very seriously; so do the unions and the National Asthma Campaign. Regulations exist and compensation is available. Yet there is surprising ignorance amongst employers. In a survey of medium to small businesses where there was a risk of occupational asthma, only one in five had introduced protective measures. The degree of awareness of the problem was highest in paint spraying operators and lowest in bakers and printers. Clearly there is much unrealized potential for prevention in industry.

Sometimes an industrial process has its impact on the public at large, and hence the asthmatics within that population. Factories must beware of spewing out effluent containing allergens, or of piling up raw materials where they are exposed to wind and weather, as in the Barcelona soya bean epidemics. These Spanish asthmatics were upset by the soya bean dust they breathed in, and developed IgE antibodies to soya. Yet as far as we can tell, they could eat soya bean products without ill effects. The idea that asthma commonly results from food allergy is false. Yet there are special circumstances where what an asthmatic eats or drinks is crucially important and these must now be mentioned.

## Food and drink

'The food should be light and easy of digestion: ripe fruits baked, boiled, or roasted are very proper, but strong liquors of all kinds especially beer or ale are hurtful. If any supper be taken it should be very light'. This advice was given to asthmatics by John Wesley in his book *Primitive Physick* published in 1747. Though questions are often raised about diet by asthmatics, there are relatively few instances where specific adjustments make much difference. There are two general rules. First, large meals filling the stomach embarrass the breathing by pressing on the diaphragm. Secondly, every effort should be made to avoid being overweight. Excess weight has to be carried, and the lungs have to provide the oxygen for energy expenditure. So the overweight asthmatic will be relatively more disabled than the asthmatic who keeps slim.

Beyond these general considerations is the question of food intolerance. Asthma is much more likely to be due to something that is inhaled into the lungs, rather than something swallowed. Yet the complaint that asthma follows soon after some particular food or drink is not uncommon.

In some instances a genuine, probably atopic, allergy is involved. The wheezing comes on within 10–15 minutes. Skin prick tests to the food or drink may be positive. Foods that can do this are cheese, fish, nuts, and fruits. This asthma is rather more likely to be accompanied by allergic symptoms elsewhere, as might be expected when the allergen must be taken into the stomach and absorbed. There may be stomach upset, with nausea, sickness, cramping pains, or an explosive diarrhoea. There may be swelling of the lips and tongue and the soft tissues of the mouth. There may be an itchy rash on the skin of the face, trunk, or limbs. All indicate that an allergen has been absorbed and distributed to all parts of the body. Food allergies can be manifested in one of these ways alone, or several features may appear together.

Once a food allergy is recognized it is easy enough to avoid. If a common ingredient seems implicated or several foods are involved then organizing an acceptable and nourishing diet might be a problem. If food allergies seem to be an important trigger factor, then the help of a dietician can be sought.

There can be ingredients added to certain foods and drinks that are capable of initiating wheezing in a few asthmatics. Of particular importance is sodium metabisulphite which causes asthma by giving off sulphur dioxide. It is used as a preservative in prepared meats, salads, and certain drinks, especially synthetic orange drinks, some wines, and beers. Alcoholic beverages feature all too frequently in the list of triggers for asthma. The alcohol itself is not at fault, but rather the additional components that give a drink its distinctive flavour or act as preservatives. Whatever the cause, sensitivity to alcoholic drinks can be one of the more annoying features of asthma.

## Medicines which can cause asthma

There are yet other things we swallow besides food and drink which are capable of triggering asthma, in particular medicines, such as aspirin (and similar pain killers) and the beta-blockers. The effects of these medicines were described earlier. It is best for asthmatics to avoid them all.

## Modifying allergic responsiveness

The best recognized way of protecting ourselves against illness is by vaccination. This technique was devised by Jenner for protection against smallpox. It used a closely related but harmless virus, vaccinia—hence the name. When applied to other infectious diseases, this process is generally now called immunization. It seems strange that such an approach should be tried for an allergic condition like asthma, but it has been. Before allergy as such was clearly described, Noon in 1911, thinking that pollen hay fever was due to a poison (or toxin) given off by the pollen, argued that if anti-toxin could be developed in the body, then the hay fever could be treated. This he hoped to achieve by injecting first very dilute and then increasingly concentrated solutions prepared from extracts of grass pollen. It appeared to be effective and later the same year Freeman first reported that asthma accompanying summer hay fever could also be helped by this treatment.

Though it later became clear that toxins were not implicated in hay fever or asthma, allergists persisted in using these injections. The technique is known as hyposensitization (not desensitization as it is often incorrectly named). It is extensively employed by specialists in allergy particularly in North America, but regarded with scepticism by others, especially physicians in Britain. For a method of treatment introduced so long ago, it is surprising and even reprehensible that there is so much doubt as at present exists about its efficacy.

In recent years the theoretical background for giving these injections has been questioned and explored. They do appear to modify allergic responsiveness. After a series of hyposensitizing injections, less of the allergy antibody IgE is produced during the pollen season and sensitivity to histamine is reduced. But are these changes accompanied by any benefit to the patient? Leaving aside asthma for a moment, there does seem reasonable evidence that hyposensitizing injections given in late winter do benefit grass hay fever and ragweed sufferers the following summer. A single set of injections will not give much 'carry-over' effect in the following season and injections have to be repeated. After several years, however, it is difficult to decide whether any relief is due directly to the injections or to the spontaneous recovery which is such a feature of summer seasonal nose allergies.

What of asthma? Here the picture is far from clear. Pollen asthma may appear to improve together with the hay fever but it may not, and asthmatic symptoms at other times of the year will be uninfluenced.

There should be a future for hyposensitization. It is effective for bee and wasp sting allergy for which highly purified allergens are available. Unfortunately an attempt to prepare similarly purified antigens for the house dust mite, produced such a powerful agent that serious allergic reactions, even deaths, were the result. This led to severe restrictions being placed on the administration of these injections in the UK so that they are now rarely given. This setback has, however, encouraged further research which promises to define more precisely what these injections do and so hopefully lead in the end to a safer and more effective form of hyposensitization treatment for allergy.

Hyposensitization is the only technique in current use that might modify allergic responsiveness. Research into the genetic basis of allergy may well lead to other approaches. Finding out even more about how the immune system behaves may, too, result in novel methods of modifying the body's responses not only to allergens, but also to infections and even other triggers of asthma.

# 15 *Patterns of care*

Asthma is pre-eminently a condition which can be managed by the patient (or by parents) under the guidance of a family doctor. Being a common disorder every family doctor will have experience in the care of asthma. Though much remains to be learned about the intimate mechanisms responsible for asthmatic wheezing, there is enough information available for every doctor to understand the principles of management. Furthermore, he should be able to tell the story of asthma sufficiently simply to enable his patients to undertake the day-to-day management of their own condition with confidence.

## Community based care

It is the family doctor who will first make the diagnosis. It is he who will distinguish asthma from wheezy bronchitis. He will be able to judge the importance of allergic triggers and emotional stresses. Inherited and environmental influences will be apparent to him because of his knowledge of the patient's family background. He will initiate treatment, preferably by inhaler. He will be the one to demonstrate its use, to ensure that each patient has the technique mastered. He will explain how and when the inhaler is to be used: whether it is to be just for the occasional wheeze: whether it is to be used prophylactically or regularly.

Family doctors will appreciate the principles on which therapy is based and will prescribe bronchodilators, DSCG, and steroid inhalers as appropriate. Asthmatics requiring more than just bronchodilators will initially require regular visits to the surgery. But a pattern of less frequent attendances is all that will be necessary when the use of these therapies has been established.

For sharp episodes of wheezing the family doctor will leave instructions about increasing medication. For those of his patients using corticosteroid therapy either intermittently or regularly, these instructions are likely to be fairly explicit, and he will most likely ask to be told when an increase in treatment has become necessary.

## Asthma clinics

Over recent years an increasing number of family doctors have been organizing special care programmes for their asthmatics. It is becoming obvious that regular check-ups to ensure that treatment is being effective are a safer way of managing asthma than a sequence of emergency visits to treat each crisis as it arises. Increasingly practice nurses take a special interest in asthmatics. Either at routine surgeries or at a special clinic, the nurse can carry out routine tasks like noting symptoms, recording the peak expiratory flow rate, checking inhaler technique, and making sure the use of the various treatments is understood. The nurse often has more time than the doctor and patients may find it easier to relate to a nurse. Such a delegation of duties requires close collaboration between the doctor and nurse. It is of paramount importance that such nurses are properly trained. The Asthma Training Centre in Stratford-on-Avon has pioneered the training of practice nurses and those who have the Centre's diploma work to a high standard. There is every hope that these community-based asthma clinics will improve the overall care of asthmatics.

A survey of community asthma clinics was carried out in 1993. All family doctors in the UK were sent a questionnaire. Replies came back from 30%, three-quarters of whom were running clinics. Most were in larger group practices and in nearly half, nurses ran these clinics by themselves. What, one wonders, is happening in the remaining 70% of practices. Subsidiary information suggests these are less likely to be running clinics. The crucial question of how effective these clinics are in improving the lot of asthmatics has yet to be answered satisfactorily. There seems intrinsic worth in tackling sensibly the care of asthma, but the best way to do this is likely to emerge as we gain experience. Targetting specific groups is one way ahead. This has been tried successfully for children and for those defined as 'at risk'.

## Self-management plans

Collaboration in asthma care not only involves doctors and nurses working together: it creates a partnership with patients and parents as well.

All asthmatics shoulder some responsibility for their own care. It may be nothing more than deciding to take two puffs from a bronchodilator inhaler when their chest is tight. Even at this

NATIONAL **ASTHMA** CAMPAIGN
*getting your breath back*

Name _____

Best peak flow _____

| | Peak Flow | Treatment |
|---|---|---|
| **1** | | Continue regular treatment |
| **2** | | Increase dose of |
| **3** | | Start oral steroids and ring doctor |
| **4** | | Call emergency medical help |

Asthma Helpline 0345 01 02 03, Monday to Friday, 9am to 9pm

| | Symptoms | Treatment |
|---|---|---|
| **1** | Asthma under control | Continue regular treatment |
| **2** | Getting a cold or waking with asthma at night | Increase dose of |
| **3** | Increasing breathlessness or poor response to | Start oral steroids and ring doctor |
| **4** | Severe attack | Call emergency medical help |

Issued by _____  Date _____

National Asthma Campaign is a registered charity, number 802364

The National Asthma Campaign asthma management credit card.

level they have to make a choice, and decide whether two puffs is enough and what to do if that doesn't work. Taking responsibility entails having some base of knowledge about asthma, some skills in handling treatment. It involves planning ahead, working things out beforehand. This is where a structured self-management plan written down in conjunction with the clinic nurse or doctor becomes invaluable.

Cards are available on which the plan can be set down. Some

of the best of these have been produced by the National Asthma Campaign. They include a note of what treatment should be taken regularly, but their great importance lies in suggesting what to do if the asthma is not effectively controlled on that regular treatment. Size is a problem and for those whose asthma is relatively straight-forward, a self-management plan has been condensed into the size of a 'credit card'.

The capricious way in which asthma catches the patient unawares and produces a sharp attack of wheezing which may settle spontaneously or may progress to a more prolonged attack, very often leads to the question: 'When do I call the doctor?' The problems of one patient are never quite the same as those of another. Despite this general guidelines are essential, since for a condition that is as treatable as asthma, there are still too many hospital admissions and even deaths.

There are several situations for which guidelines are needed: for example a sudden sharp increase in symptoms and a slow deterioration over a few days. Most asthmatics expect a certain amount of variability in wheezing from moment to moment, or day to day and so can recognize the sudden change that heralds a sharp attack. A recurrence of night-time awakening with cough or wheezing, or a failure of usually successful remedies to be effective are two signals that an attack is building up. Increasingly the peak flow machine is being used at home by asthmatics to monitor progress. Different criteria of change will apply to different patients: it may be a sudden fall in peak flow by a specific amount, a drop below a critical level, or the failure of peak flow to rise in the evening above the figure obtained in the morning.

These recognizable signs of impending trouble need to be incor-porated into a plan. So the plan might describe action to be taken 'for sudden chest tightness, breathlessness or wheeze'. This could be a certain dose of bronchodilator using a certain device. And there would be instructions 'if that does not give relief, then take . . .'.

A slower deterioration, a recurrence of nocturnal awakening previ-ously abolished, the onset of a chesty cold, or a fall in peak flow on one or more occasions by a specified amount or percentage: these all might be combatted by a recommended change in regular maintenance treatment or starting steroids in some form.

The essence of such plans is that they are tailor-made for an

## Zone 1

**Your asthma is under control if:**

- Your peak flow readings are above

  _____
  and
- it does not disturb your sleep
  and
- it does not restrict your activities

### Action

**Continue your normal medicines**

## Zone 2

(Your doctor or nurse may decide not to use this zone)

**Your asthma is getting worse if:**

- Your peak flow readings have fallen to between

  _____
  and _____
- You are needing to use your

  (reliever inhaler) more than usual
- You are waking at night with asthma symptoms

### Action

- **Increase your**

  _____
  (preventer inhaler) to

  _____
- **Continue to take your**

  (reliever inhaler) to relieve your asthma symptoms

---

## Zone 3

**Your asthma is severe if:**

- Your peak flow readings have fallen to between

  _____
  and
  _____
- You are getting increasingly breathless
- You are needing to use your

  (reliever inhaler) every

  _____ hours or more often

### Action

**Ring your doctor or nurse**

- Take _____ prednisolone (steroid) tablets (_____ mg each) and then

  _____

  _____
- Discuss with your doctor how to stop taking the tablets
- Continue to take your

  _____
  (reliever and preventer inhalers) as required

## Zone 4

**Medical alert/emergency if:**

- Your peak flow readings have fallen to below
- You continue to get worse

**Do not be afraid of causing a fuss. Your doctor will want to see you urgently.**

### Action

**Get help immediately**

- Ring your doctor immediately

  (Telephone _____)
  or call an ambulance
- Take _____ prednisolone (steroid) tablets (_____ mg each) immediately
- Continue to take your

  _____
  (reliever inhaler) as needed

Self-management instructions based on a 'zone' plan.

individual, written down, but subject always to revision in the light of experience. An example of one such plan is shown. Parents will hold and follow the plans devised for young children, and accessory cards with relevant instructions have been produced for use by the child's teacher at school.

## The acute attack

Even with the very best of care and despite carefully designed management plans, asthma sometimes gets out of control.

### Helping the asthmatic through an attack

'What should I do when he can't get his breath?' asks the mother of an asthmatic child. 'All I could do was to stand by helpless' says the boss whose secretary had an attack of asthma. Perhaps the first rule is to remain calm yourself. Wheezing provokes anxiety and no asthmatic likes being at the mercy of his asthma. If your child, friend, or partner senses that you are panicking, that you are uncertain what to do, their anxiety will be compounded.

Ensure that whatever medicines have been advised for an attack are taken properly. Sometimes it is impossible for the asthmatic to get an effective breath in so that even the dry powder devices can't be easily used. Spacers are an ideal answer. A makeshift spacer can be devised by forcing a hole in the bottom of a plastic polythene coffee cup. Nebulizers are obviously ideal if they are available. In the absence of any of these devices, it is important that the simple pressurized inhaler is used as effectively as possible and if the asthmatic is too distraught to synchronize the firing of the inhaler, then whoever is helping in the attack can do that, ensuring that they fire the inhaler on a breath in.

Apart from taking the medication, make sure that the asthmatic is comfortable in the attack: sitting in a chair or on the edge of a bed, often leaning forward slightly. Encourage relaxation and slow breathing. With a child do something to occupy his mind. What you choose depends on your child—TV, a record, a story read aloud, a puzzle. Adults more often just want to be quiet. All the time, emphasis will be on an outward quiet confidence and an inward alertness on the part of the carer. Calm does not mean carelessness, for there are signs to look for that suggest whether or not the doctor should be called.

---

## When to call for help in the acute attack

- Breathlessness severe enough to confine to bed or chair
- Inability to talk in complete sentences
- Too breathless to feed (child)
- Failure of emergency relief medicine to give benefit (bronchodilator e.g. Ventolin)

If you are able to make measurements:
- peak flow rate down to half best (or predicted) value after using bronchodilator

---

## Calling the doctor

If these measures do not result in the attack abating quickly, then do not hesitate to call for help. A family doctor visiting an asthmatic in a sharp attack at home will need to satisfy himself that his patient has correctly taken prescribed bronchodilators. If these have failed to abate the attack, a nebulizer will deliver that larger dose of inhaled bronchodilator that is needed for the sharp attack. If experience suggests that a course of steroids is likely to be necessary, the doctor will possibly start this with an injection of hydrocortisone or alternatively give a supply of prednisolone tablets. Observation over about half an hour will generally be sufficient to judge whether the attack is settling. About one in ten acute attacks of asthma seen in this way at home do not settle, and hospital admission becomes necessary.

## Hospital care

### Emergency admission

The acutely ill patient can expect to be the centre of attention on arrival in hospital. Assessment will be telescoped into a few minutes with the details omitted. Oxygen is likely to be given through a mask and nebulized bronchodilators are the rule. Steroids will be given, either prednisolone by mouth, or injected hydrocortisone. A drip line may be fed into a vein for giving further treatment. Progress over the first few hours will be watched closely. Pulse rate, blood pressure, peak expiratory flow will be recorded, and the treatment schedule adjusted accordingly. Physiotherapists may be called in to help with coughing and relaxation.

Rarely, the immediate medication does not bring relief and the laboured breathing brings fatigue and exhaustion with the danger that breathing movement will become inadequate. Not only is oxygenation impaired but the carbon dioxide that should be eliminated by the lungs is retained in the body. This causes clouding of consciousness and eventual coma. Resort is made at this stage to artificial ventilation. The number of times this is required will not be more than a handful throughout a whole county each year—but when judiciously and appropriately applied, it is life saving.

## The hospital out-patients

While the major responsibility for the care of asthma in the community rests with the family doctor, asthma is only one of a legion of problems with which he has to deal. He cannot be expected to have at his fingertips knowledge of every facet of the diagnosis and management of a single problem. So he may turn to the hospital physician. He may choose to refer the asthmatic to a hospital out-patient department for a variety of reasons. There may be some question mark over the diagnosis. Is this really asthma? Have I missed an allergy? In the adult, how much is smoking contributing? Or it may be that he is clear about the diagnosis and wants the reassurance of a specialist's opinion: perhaps more often wants that reassurance for the patient's sake, or with children for the parents' sake. Fashions in treatment are constantly changing: new therapies are introduced. He may not be sure that he is using precisely the correct therapy for this particular asthmatic nor that he is using the correct dosage for maximal effect: so he asks for advice.

Asthmatic patients may be seen in a general medical clinic where the physician or paediatrician will have broadly based skills covering a wide range of medical problems. Increasingly the physician will be one with a special interest in chest problems who may hold specialized clinics devoted to asthma.

A detailed history and physical examination are essential parts of the hospital assessment and so is some sort of objective measurement of lung function. If at the time of clinic attendance some asthma is present, the degree to which this can be immediately reversed with a bronchodilator aerosol will probably be checked. If there is no wheeze, more often in children, an immediate exercise test might be carried out to see if wheezing develops after exertion. Depending on a whole host

| | Days | | | | | | | Leave this column blank |
|---|---|---|---|---|---|---|---|---|
| Date of day of start    /    / **198** | 1 | 2 | 3 | 4 | 5 | 6 | 7 | |
| **(1) Night** | | | | | | | | |
| Good night                                    0<br>Woken once by asthma                  1<br>Woken × 2–3 because of asthma   2<br>Bad night, awake most of time       3 | | | | | | | | |
| **(2) Day** | | | | | | | | |
| Symptom free                          0<br>Wheezy for an hour or two      1<br>Wheezy for much of the day   2<br>Wheezy all day                          3 | | | | | | | | |
| **(3) Peak flow gauge readings**<br>On waking in morning | | | | | | | | |
| About 6 p.m. | | | | | | | | |
| **(4) Drugs in 24 hrs.** | | | | | | | | |
| Intal: no. of capsules inhaled | | | | | | | | |
| Bronchodilator: no. of puffs<br>(_____) | | | | | | | | |
| Steroid aerosol: no. of puffs<br>(_____) | | | | | | | | |
| Prednisone: ____total in mgs.<br>Other (specify) _____ | | | | | | | | |
| **(5) Comments**<br>Report anything unusual<br>e.g. a cold | | | | | | | | |

A typical diary card.

of circumstances, other tests might be asked for: some of which will be directed towards seeking the cause—or causes of the asthma.

The outcome of such a visit will vary according to the needs of the patient. Some advice may be given about lifestyle, about the avoidance of allergens, about stopping smoking, about occupation. The physician may ask the asthmatic to chart day-by-day fluctuations in the amount of asthma he experiences by using a diary card. These estimations of symptoms will be accompanied by recordings of lung function at home with the portable peak flow machine. The outcome of such a visit will vary, partly with the requirements of the patient, partly with the approach of the physician, partly with the relationship between that physician and the patient's general practitioner. In a few instances especially where there are complex features in the causation of the asthma, where the condition has become chronic, where conventional treatment has been tried and failed, where there are other diseases complicating the issue, the family doctor will ask the hospital to keep a regular check on an asthmatic. In others the issues will be simply resolved and the patient can be discharged from hospital surveillance and returned to the supervision of the community asthma clinic.

## Investigation and research

The investigation of mechanisms in asthma can take several forms. Sophisticated lung function testing can indicate the degree and extent of the airways' narrowing. Agents likely to provoke asthma may be tested for their effect on the airways' narrowing. This could be followed by evaluating therapeutic drugs for their ability to protect against such a challenge.

The hinterland between clinical management and research becomes blurred when mechanisms are being investigated or new drugs evaluated. The results will be pertinent to the management of the specific individual, but they also add to the body of information about mechanisms and therapy that will forward research in asthma. It should no longer be necessary for anyone to fear being a guinea pig. Safeguards are wide ranging and carried out stringently. All new drugs have been exhaustively tested in experimental animals. They will be used cautiously in humans for short periods, before long-term trials in patients are undertaken. Careful blood checks are carried out and frequent clinical assessments made.

What questions are being asked in asthma research? A great deal of effort is expended in trying to discern the details of mechanisms. Of the major trigger factors, much is known about allergy, but the early atopic allergic reaction seems little in evidence in clinical asthma. Late reactions would seem to explain the clinical pattern of asthma much more satisfactorily and a great deal is now known about what is going on in the airways during these reactions. Much mystery still surrounds the way in which infections trigger asthma and this field would seem to be one in which there is most to be learned. The importance of psychological triggers will continue to be debated for many years. If suggestion has such a powerful effect as that apparent in anecdotal observations and some carefully conducted studies, then the means of harnessing it and putting it to use need to be explored. It is becoming clear that irritability of the airways is the common underlying defect in all asthma, but much has yet to be learned about it. The problem of heredity in allergy and asthma is on the threshold of being solved and its relevance in a therapeutic sense is wide open. New therapies are continually being put forward by the pharmaceutical companies. They require evaluation in clinical asthma. Some, like DSCG, contribute considerably to understanding the ways in which asthmatic wheezing is brought about.

# 16  *Living with asthma*

In the past, asthma was a condition really only known about because of the attacks it produced. It was assumed that once the attack was over, you no longer needed to think about the asthma. As we have seen, that has now changed. Asthma is a condition that we know is present between attacks but we know too that with modern treatment it can be controlled. Sometimes asthma does completely go away so that regular treatment is not needed, and whilst there is always a chance that it will come back, a lot of people are able to say that they used to have asthma. Despite a potential threat they can lead lives untroubled by the actuality or the thought of asthma. Others are not so fortunate and they need to live with their asthma. They have to live with the need for treatment and with the limitations that having asthma places upon their everyday lives.

## Taking the treatment

Drug companies produce very effective treatments for asthma, and doctors know how to prescribe them. But the treatment won't be effective, unless the asthmatic actually takes it as recommended. Our approach to any sort of treatment is conditioned by our upbringing, our attitudes, and the way taking that treatment is presented to us. There is always a conflict between the desire to do the best we can for ourselves and our children by taking the treatment regularly and the wish to be free of the encumbrance of always having to remember to take that treatment. And we get conflicting advice. One hopes this does not come from the profession, although there are some uncertainties about which treatment should be used and when. It is rather more likely to come from our family, our friends, our workmates, the articles we read in magazines, and the documentaries we see on television. These tend to give a biased view and it is not always the same bias, so we are confused. Some of the uncertainty about asthma treatment arises because of potential side effects. Side effects from asthma treatment are relatively few. There are some real side effects, as we showed in an earlier chapter, which we must rightly be aware of, but it is important that we do not fail to take effective treatment just because of the fear of possible, or even imagined, side effects.

With many asthmatics correct treatment in doses that do not cause side effects will give virtually complete control of their asthma, and that is indeed the aim of modern treatment. Having said that, when questioned, many asthmatics obviously have limitations to their lifestyle as a result of their asthma. It may be that they recognize that certain conditions, fumes, or dusts trigger off their asthma and so adapt their lives in order to avoid them. This may mean not having pets at home, it may mean avoiding going into smoky pubs, it may mean changing leisure activities.

## Schooling

The parents of an asthmatic child face decisions in relation to school. It is usually the immediate daily decision as to whether your child is well enough to go to school on a given day. It is easy enough to judge when you have had a fretful night and there is obvious wheezing, but it is not always easy to set these objective features against the whims and manipulations of your child. Maybe homework hasn't been finished or there is a lesson that is disliked. Or maybe you are out at work and you wonder who on earth is going to look after your child if he or she does not go to school. You may be afraid too that the teachers won't allow medication to be used as freely as you would like. Education of school teachers is actively going on and one hopes that this is a thing of the past.

## Exercise and sport

Many asthmatics become frustrated because they cannot participate in sport as much as they would like to. It is important to realize that exercise is not harmful to the asthmatic. Indeed physical fitness is beneficial to the asthmatic as it is to anyone else. The special problem of exercise-induced asthma needs to be faced and appropriate medication taken before exercise, either a bronchodilator or sodium cromoglycate. If it is a question of adapting sporting activity, it is worth remembering that athletic sports and games such as tennis which necessitate a degree of continuous activity are less well tolerated than games such as football or cricket in which there are short bursts of activity punctuated by spells of relative inactivity. Most asthmatics enjoy swimming in which water takes the weight of the body. Indeed Olympic medals have been won for swimming by asthmatics.

## Occupation

For the majority of asthmatics there needs to be little restriction on occupation but it is important that if specific allergies are known to exist then an occupation exposing the asthmatic to these allergens is obviously to be avoided. So those sensitive to dog hair should not become kennel maids: those sensitive to pollen should not become gardeners and specific occupational hazards such as those referred to in Chapter 8 should also be avoided.

## Disability

For those who have regular or repeated symptoms, there is a general effect on lifestyle. Repeatedly waking up at night, disturbs sleep and means being tired during the day. Those who are permanently short of breath, think about where they are going to park the car or how far they have to walk. Fortunately very few asthmatics become permanently disabled. Central to determining disability is the question of dependency. The degree to which shortness of breath interferes with daily life will depend very much on personal circumstances. A car copes with mobility problems but only for those who can afford it. A farm worker may well have to give up his job because of his asthma whereas the housewife will carry on, perhaps with help. Those who are anxious or obsessional will cope less well with shortness of breath than the more phlegmatic. With asthma these problems only reach bothersome proportions in a few individuals with chronic and continuous symptoms. Rather more asthmatics have to face the somewhat different problem of the acute attack. This introduces the disability of uncertainty, which is a consequence of unpredictable interference by an attack with daily routine.

As with all chronic illness those who have constant symptoms from their asthma, despite all that modern treatment can do, need sympathy and understanding not only for its own sake but for the way in which they can help the asthmatic to cope with a restricted way of life.

## Beyond drug therapy

Most asthmatics and their carers would prefer to be free of the encumbrance and necessity of taking medication. Many are anxious about side effects. So what can asthmatics do to help themselves and how can those who look after them collaborate.

The first, and perhaps the most obvious, is allergen avoidance. This we have already discussed in some detail (Chapter 13). Clearly there are important ways in which allergic and occupational triggers for asthma can be reduced. Such an approach will only apply where an obvious external trigger is implicated. But there are a whole host of other measures from relaxation to complementary medicine that we need to think about. But first, one golden rule. Whilst many of these measures may help, they should not be used as an alternative to conventional treatment. So NEVER stop asthma medications suddenly. This can lead to a sharp attack. On the other hand, there is every reason to gradually reduce the amount of medication under medical supervision so that minimum doses can be reached which keep the asthma under control.

## Relaxation and breathing exercises

The fear engendered by the approach, or the actual experience, of an attack of asthma causes tension. This tension is felt in the muscles around the neck, shoulders, and even in the arms and trunk. Whether it can also be reflected in tension in the muscles around the airways is not certain. Increasing tension does seem to escalate the distress caused by an asthma attack; and the relaxation of tension, to lessen it. Awareness of tension is the first step to relieving it. Techniques of relaxation learned when the asthma is quiescent can be brought into use when an attack of wheezing develops. They enable the asthmatic, in some indefinable way, to cope with the attack.

The most sophisticated use of relaxation and muscle control is in yoga. For those versed in these techniques, or willing and able to learn them, they offer an excellent way of providing the relief from tension in an asthmatic attack, that will enable medications to have their optimal effect. There is even a suggestion that yoga exercises actually make the airways a little less twitchy.

Beyond simple relaxation comes the question of breathing exercises. This is a controversial area in the treatment of chest conditions. Though widely used for many decades, breathing exercises have only recently become the subject of scientific scrutiny.

It is not possible voluntarily to influence the muscles of the air passages themselves. We can, on the other hand, exercise some control over the muscles which surround the chest and so move the lungs. So it is possible to alter the rate of breathing, the depth of breathing, and the relative contributions of various muscle groups to the movement of the chest. Even so, voluntary control is restricted by the requirement to breathe in through the lungs the amount of oxygen needed by the body.

Sitting still we naturally breathe about 10–12 times a minute. Breathing is faster when exercising, slower when sleeping. The rate of breathing is also capable of internal adjustment in the face of obstacles placed in the way of the free flow of air in and out of the lungs. In asthma the airways are narrowed. A moment's thought will reveal that more effort is going to be required to force air quickly through a narrow tube than to blow gently and slowly. It will thus be more economical of effort to breathe slowly and deeply through narrowed airways than it will be to breathe rapidly and shallowly. A slow breathing pattern with the time taken to breathe out, set at twice that to breathe in, is taught in yoga. Some asthmatics find that they adopt this pattern naturally. Others, perhaps because of a sense of panic, seem to breathe more quickly than is really necessary, and become more distressed. The message to the asthmatic, then, is to breathe slowly. A word of caution must be added. Slow breaths can become deep breaths, and deep breathing may lead to overbreathing. This will cause dizziness and tingling in the fingers, and can even make the asthma worse. So it is to be avoided.

It was once commonly taught that asthmatics should empty their lungs with each breath. This encourages a forcing of the air out, and compression of the lungs to a smaller size than they would reach at the end of a natural breath. This is wrong. It is wrong because it encourages not only compression of the lungs but compression, too, of the airways themselves, the very airways through which it is hoped to empty the lungs. Relief will come if breathing is controlled at a slow rate with gentle breathing-out, allowing the lungs to relax down to a natural resting position but not forcing them beyond that.

There is agreement that relaxation and slow breathing are both beneficial and sound, in a scientific sense. Controversy surrounds the various techniques which claim to make it possible to move one part of the chest more than another.

Conscious control over one group of muscles rather than another has been attempted, but requires training and there is no evidence that a learned pattern can be transmitted into the unconscious control of natural breathing. It must be used consciously and deliberately when it is required.

Emphasis is sometimes given to what has been called diaphragmatic breathing. As the diaphragm moves downwards during breathing in, it compresses the contents of the abdomen. It is natural for the muscles of the front wall of the abdomen to relax as this happens. Sometimes in asthma, this natural relaxation does not occur and these muscles may even be tightened in common with the tension developed in muscles elsewhere. This could restrict the downward movement of the diaphragm. The description 'diaphragmatic breathing' is given to the techniques for increasing awareness of the movement of the front of the abdomen, so that the downward movement of the diaphragm can proceed unimpeded. Training will ensure that this pattern is maintained when wheezing develops, and many asthmatics find it beneficial.

## Hypnosis

This takes the principle of relaxation a step further. In Chapter 6 some studies were mentioned in which inert salt solutions could be made to cause airways' narrowing or relaxation, demonstrating that suggestion can influence the airways. It seems, also, that it can influence allergic responses. Under hypnosis, skin prick tests for atopic allergy were rendered negative in one arm, but not in the other, which it was suggested, would react normally.

Some physicians carry out hypnosis treatment for asthma. Initially they use hypnosis by the physician, but try to teach autohypnosis as soon as possible. This means that the patient can hypnotize himself for 15–30 minutes each day at home, the idea being to reinforce the therapeutic suggestions previously given by the doctor. Safeguards are built in against the fear of helplessness in alarming situations, against children demonstrating their skills at school, and against staying hypnotized for too long. During a year's observation the amount of asthma in a group of patients treated with hypnosis was reduced by one-third. A control group given simple relaxation also improved greatly and not until 8 months of treatment had been carried out did the hypnosis group fare better than the controls.

The questions that need answering about hypnosis are several. Does the recorded freedom from asthma go along with better lung function? If not, then is the apparent unawareness by the patient of the degree

of asthma helpful or harmful? The shortness of breath experienced by
the asthmatic can be very alarming; to reduce his awareness of this
might well help him to cope more easily with everyday life. On the
other hand, if it made him oblivious to a serious deterioration in his
asthma, it would be potentially dangerous.

If long-term improvement can be substantiated it might well be
questioned whether it is all worthwhile when seen in relation to
the wide variety of pharmacological agents now available. A positive
answer would perhaps only be given for the chronic asthmatic in whom
the time and effort involved in organizing hypnosis is to be set against
the potential hazards of steroid therapy.

## Psychotherapy

Any physician, by taking a careful history and listening sympatheti-
cally to an asthmatic patient's problems will be able to provide
sufficient psychotherapy to alleviate much of the anxiety experienced by the average asthmatic. Misunderstanding is a potent source
of anxiety in asthma as in other illnesses. A clear explanation of
the mechanisms leading to episodes of asthma and the ways of
most easily coping with attacks, are simple and important tools
that any physician can use to help the asthmatic. A common-sense
approach to everyday problems that are providing stress, perhaps
with the help of a social worker, can deal with a vast majority of
problems.

On a more specific plane, it is important that a truly depressive
illness be identified, for the appropriate treatment of this can lead
to the asthma once more becoming manageable. Psychotherapy, as
such, is reserved for the very few patients with complex psychological
problems. Its design is usually the simple one of reducing anxiety
and tension. It requires time and dedication on the parts of both
the patient and the doctor, perhaps most of all in techniques which
attempt to 'desensitize' the asthmatic to stressful circumstances. In the
quiet atmosphere of the clinic, the psychotherapist suggests in a limited
way the stressful psychological circumstances that are thought to be
responsible for a patient's asthma. By applying relaxation techniques,
the asthmatic can be made to accept a small degree of stress without
becoming wheezy. Over weeks or months, the degree of stress
is gradually increased and the relaxation reinforced until finally it
should be possible for the asthmatic to experience without trouble

a degree of stress in real life which had previously caused asthmatic wheezing.

## Acupuncture

The Chinese discovered the first bronchodilator, ephedrine, but it took 4000 years for the West to realize its worth. They also discovered acupuncture but the first serious analyses of its value have only recently been carried out. In asthma there is now good evidence that acupuncture can relax the airways. The effect seems immediate and short-lived, rather like that to be expected from a bronchodilator. Carefully controlled studies have shown unequivocally that needling of the '*Din Chuan*' spot, just below the back of the neck, brings some relief to asthmatic wheezing, whereas the same procedure applied to non-specific points on the body has no effect. This observation could have important implications for research into the mechanisms of asthma. It could also form the basis for treatment in a few individuals, but the ease and simplicity of administration of a bronchodilator means that acupuncture will never be the first-line treatment for asthma.

The evidence that acupuncture given repeatedly can alter the course of asthma is far less clear cut. Anecdotal observations report both improvement in lung function and a diminution in the requirements for inhalers. Formal trials are less convincing, and bedevilled by the problems of finding a suitable 'control' treatment against which the acupuncture can be judged.

## Homeopathy

The principles that lie behind the practice of homeopathy are difficult to comprehend for those brought up on modern medical science. In practice, substances are chosen which when given in high dose seem to mimic the symptom that it is designed to treat. An exceedingly dilute solution of the substance is then made and administered as the homeopathic medicine. Various trials in a whole variety of conditions have been carried out. As far as asthma is concerned there is only one properly conducted study to have shown any benefit. Symptoms did improve, and somewhat less inhaler treatment was used, but lung function did not alter. The case for homeopathy in asthma is unproven. More careful trials will be needed to decide for certain one way or the other.

## *Ionizers*

Ions are minute atmospheric particles carrying an electrical charge either positive or negative. Normally there are very few of these in the atmosphere. A few more arise with intense ultraviolet light from a scorching sun or after an electrical storm. In a closed room with little change of air, the ion content will drop to almost imperceptible levels.

Very wide-ranging claims are made for the effects of ions on man. It is suggested that the lethargy that overpowers the average office worker towards the end of the day is due to lack of ions. A study in a Swiss bank claimed that by creating a negatively charged atmosphere, workers not only became more efficient but that they also lost less time from work on account of respiratory illness.

How far can these claims be substantiated in respect of asthma? Sadly it seems not very far. There is anecdotal support for benefit, and one good study showing some protection against exercise-induced asthma in children from breathing negatively charged ions. Most investigations, however, have failed to substantiate claims made for ionizers in asthma.

## *National Asthma Campaign*

Great benefit can come from the formation of a charity which concerns itself with a particular medical condition. The two great cancer charities, the Cancer Research Campaign and the Imperial Cancer Research Fund were both formed in the early years of this century and are still going strong. Of others, the Diabetic Association is well known. It started in the 1930s at about the time insulin became available, and diabetics needed to learn how to give injections to themselves. Between these came the first asthma charity, the Asthma Research Council which was founded in 1927. Little was known about asthma at the time. Misconceptions were rife and treatment was pretty rudimentary. Research was considered the priority and so began the long haul that eventually led up to our present day understanding of the nature and treatment of asthma.

As we noted earlier, the 1960s and 1970s saw dramatic advances in the treatment available for asthmatics. The concept of taking medicine by inhalation was introduced. This brought great benefits but it also created problems. Just as diabetic patients had needed help in taking their injections, so asthmatic patients needed help and advice on taking their inhalers if they were going to obtain maximum benefit from them. This required a different slant in the charitable approach to asthma, one directed towards the patient's personal needs rather than research into the disease itself. Such endeavours began first in New Zealand and Australia. Inspired by these organizations we in the UK set about forming a similar charity towards the end of the 1970s. The basis for a patients' organization already existed in the Friends of the Asthma Research Council. It was decided to use this as the nucleus for the Asthma Society which was formed in 1980.

The aims of the charity were threefold: to spread information about asthma: to provide a branch organization for helping asthmatics and to raise funds for research conducted by the Asthma Research Council. The charity found there was a large unmet need for the services it aimed to provide, especially in the areas in information and guidance. The two charities then united at the beginning of 1990, as the National Asthma Campaign.

The NAC spends 60% of its money on research—nearly 2 million pounds a year, funding projects that span every aspect of asthma. The branch network now numbers around 200. Branch activities include fundraising, swimming and other sporting activities, and a source of advice. The Campaign's pamphlets are some of the most informative available for any condition. A telephone helpline was set up in 1989. Trained nurses answer calls ranging from simple requests for information, to distressing cries for help (Tel. 0345 010203).

The charity has embraced the campaigning role embodied in its new name by tackling wider issues. The making-available of peak flow meters on prescription was a result of pressures put on the Department of Health. It has supported the pioneering work of the National Asthma Training Centre for nurses in Stratford and sponsored, with the doctors' professional body, the British Thoracic Society postgraduate lectures for doctors. A recent venture funded and coordinated through the NAC has been the creation of a UK National Asthma Task Force to which professional societies, statutory bodies, epidemiologists, clinicians, and scientists all contribute their expertise.

What can the NAC offer the asthmatics reading this book? Immediate contact for advice and help; written information to reflect on, 'branch meetings', workshops, and conferences to help you explore more about asthma; opportunities to join in fundraising; and the satisfaction of seeing donations leading to successful research results.

## Postscript

It is evident that some major changes have occurred since I first attempted to put down the facts about asthma. Asthma now has a higher profile in the eyes of both the public and the profession than ever before. Knowledge about asthma has increased immeasurably both amongst scientists and doctors and amongst patients and their carers. More asthmatics are using regular inhaled protective therapy and benefiting from the improved control this gives over their condition. Delivery systems for inhaled medicines are now much more efficient.

Yet despite all this there is no room for complacency. There is no true cure for asthma. Possible ways of avoiding the trigger factors for asthma, particularly allergies, are being explored, but it would be preferable if the unnatural reactivity of the airways could be so corrected that the restriction needed for effective avoidance became unnecessary. Tried and tested treatment schemes for acute asthma have been widely endorsed and put into practice, but deaths from asthma still occur. Agreed recommendations for the management of persistent asthma have been published and publicized, but still many asthmatics lead lives of less than optimal quality because of their condition. Despite intense research, there is still much to be learned about what actually goes on in asthmatic airways. Despite multimillion pound investment on the part of the pharmaceutical industry, no new approach to the treatment of asthma has appeared which has ousted inhaled corticosteroids from the central role they have established since their introduction 30 years ago. Despite wide ranging and successful educational endeavour, there are still many crying out for a better understanding of their condition.

The present trends of an increasing prevalence of asthma and allergic disorders show no early signs of reversing, and those who research the causes of asthma will not lack work for decades to come. Since new asthmatics come with each generation, the work of trainers and educationalists will continue to be needed. Until a radically new direction for treatment is discovered, asthmatics will need sustained diligence in managing their own condition, and books on the facts about and the mysteries surrounding asthma will hopefully continue to be in demand.

# Glossary

●●●●●●●●●●●●●●●●●●●●●●●●●●●●●●●●●●●●●●●●●●●●●●●●●

*Note: items in italics are also defined in the glossary*

**acetylcholine**—a chemical that carries messages from nerves in the *parasympathetic nervous system* which make airway muscle tighten

**adrenaline**—a chemical that causes airway muscle to relax: it circulates in the blood and also carries messages in the *sympathetic nervous system*

**allergens**—particles found in the environment (dust, pollen etc.) which cause allergic reactions, such as asthma or hay fever, in susceptible people

**allergy**—a condition where an individual is unduly sensitive to *allergens*

**alveoli**—the air spaces of the lungs: air is carried to the alveoli by *bronchi* and oxygen passes across the alveolar wall into the blood

**antibiotic**—a drug which treats infection

**antibody**—a protein produced by the body's immune defences in response to contact with allergens, infections, etc.

**anticholinergic** – a *bronchodilator* that works by antagonizing the effect of *acetylcholine*

**antihistamine**—a drug which antagonizes *histamine*

**atopy**—a particular allergic condition of individuals who have asthma, eczema, rhinitis, and urticaria

**autonomic nervous system**—that part of the body's nerve network that operates involuntary muscles and glands e.g. eyes, gut, blood vessels, bronchi

**$\beta_2$ agonist**—a *bronchodilator* which acts like *adrenaline* to relax airway muscle so allowing the airway to widen

**bronchi**—the air passages inside the lungs: the smallest in size are called bronchioles

**bronchodilators**—drugs which open up narrowed *bronchi*—see also $\beta$ agonist, anticholinergic, methylxanthine

**cytokines**—chemical messengers that are involved in the inflammation found in asthmatic airways

**disodium cromoglycate (DSCG)**—a drug which protects against atopic allergy

**eczema**—an itchy red and weeping rash of the skin especially in the bends of the knees, elbows, wrists, etc. due to atopic allergy

**emphysema**—a destruction of the walls of the air spaces in the lungs (the alveoli) generally caused by smoking

**eosinophil**—one of the scavenger cells of the blood which is attracted to areas of allergic inflammation

**FEV$_1$ (forced expiratory volume in one second)**—the volume of air which can be forced out of the lungs in one second after taking a full breath in

**histamine**—a chemical which causes the airways to tighten and is released from *mast cells* during an allergic reaction

**house dust mite**—a small creature found in household dust and a very common cause of allergic reactions

**IgE**—the *antibody* produced by the body as a result of encountering an allergen, specifically one involved in atopic allergy

**lymphocytes**—key cells in the immune system which produce *antibodies* and *cytokines*

**mast cell**—a cell found in the airways to which IgE antibody attaches itself: it contains many chemicals including *histamine*

**methylxanthine**—a type of bronchodilator only available as a tablet and not as an inhaler

**parasympathetic nervous system**—part of the *autonomic nervous system* which is concerned with digestive and restorative functions

**PEFR or PEF (Peak expiratory flow rate)**—the maximum flow of air out of the lungs when air is forced out after taking a full breath in

**prednisone**—the most commonly used corticosteroid tablet for asthma

**rhinitis**—inflammation producing sneezing and running of the nose, which may be caused by allergy, as in hay fever (allergic rhinitis due to grass pollen)

**steroid aerosol**—a solution of a corticosteroid for inhaling

**sympathetic nervous system**—part of the autonomic nervous system concerned with preparation for activity

**urticaria**—an atopic allergic reaction of the skin which consists of raised itchy weals or blotches and is often due to allergy to food

# Useful addresses

## Societies: UK

National Asthma Campaign, Providence House, Providence Place, London N1 0NT (Tel: 0171 226 2260) Helpline (03454 010203)

Asthma Training Centre, Winton House, Church Street, Stratford-upon-Avon, Warwickshire, England, CV37 6HB (Tel: 01789 296974)

British Lung Foundation, 78 Hatton Gardens, London EC1N 8JR (Tel: 0171 831 5831)

National Eczema Society, 163 Eversholt Street, London NW1 1BU (Tel: 0171 388 4097)

### Abroad

Asthma Society of **Ireland**, 24 Anglesea Street, Dublin 2

Asthma Foundation of New South Wales, 82–86 Pacific Highway, St Leonards, NSW 2065 Australia
(Other states have their own AFs)

Asthma Society of **New Zealand**, PO Box 1459, Wellington, New Zealand

Asthma and Allergy Foundation, Washington DC, USA

**Canadian** Lung Association (national office), 1900 City Park Drive, Suite 508, Blair Business Park, Gloucester, Ontario, KLJ 1A3

## Businesses

Clement Clarke International Ltd, Airmed House, Edinburgh Way, Harlow, Essex CM20 2ED (Tel: 01279 414969) (peak flow meters)

Ferraris Medical Ltd, 26 Lea Valley Trading Estate, Angel Road, Edmonton, London N18 3JD (Tel: 0181 807 3636) (peak flow meters)

W L Gore & Associates, Intervent, Simpson Parkway, Kirkton Campus, Livingstone, West Lothian, Scotland (Tel: 01506 412 525) (mattress covers)

Medic Alert Foundation, 12 Bridge Wharf, 156 Caledonian Road, London N1 9UU (Tel: 0171 833 3034) (steroid warning bracelets and necklaces)

Medivac Healthcare Products Ltd, Market House, Church Street, Wilmslow, Cheshire SK9 1AU (Tel: 01625 539401) (specialized vacuum cleaners)

Medix Ltd, Medix House, Main Street, Catthorpe, Lutterworth, Leics LE17 6DB (01788 860366) (nebulizers)

Vitalograph Ltd, Maids Moreton House, Buckingham, MK18 1SW (Tel: 01280 822811) (peak flow meters)

Vorwerk (UK) Ltd, Unit A, Toutley Road, Wokingham, Berks RG11 1QN (Tel: 01734 794878)

## Complementary medicine

British Acupuncture Council, Park House, 206–8 Latimer Road, London W10 6RE (Tel: 0181 964 0222)

British Homeopathic Association, 27A Devonshire Street, London W1N 1RJ (Tel: 0171 935 2163)

Osteopathic Information Service, PO Box 2074, Reading RG1 4YR (Tel: 01734 512051)

British Chiropractic Association, 29 Whitley Street, Reading, Berks RG2 0EG (Tel: 01734 257557)

# Index

∙∙∙∙∙∙∙∙∙∙∙∙∙∙∙∙∙∙∙∙∙∙∙∙∙∙∙∙∙∙∙∙∙∙∙∙∙∙∙∙∙∙∙∙∙∙∙∙